Primary Palliative Care

Dying, death and bereavement in the community

Senic _____ _ _____ _ ___fessional Development,
Centre for _____nary Health Care Studies
and
Assistant Director, School of Postgraduate Medical Education,
University of Warwick

Foreword by

Professor Sir Kenneth Calman

Radcliffe Medical Press

Radcliffe Medical Press Ltd
18 Marcham Road
Abingdon
Oxon OX14 1AA
United Kingdom

www.radcliffe-oxford.com
The Radcliffe Medical Press electronic catalogue and online ordering facility.
Direct sales to anywhere in the world.

British Library Cataloguing in Publication Data

A catalogue record for this book is available from the British Library.

ISBN 1 85775 573 1

Typeset by Aarontype Ltd, Easton, Bristol
Printed and bound by TJ International Ltd, Padstow, Cornwall

Contents

Foreword

Primary care is at the sharp end of clinical practice. In many instances more acute work is carried on in this setting than in the hospital environment. This has put increasing pressure on the primary care team to deliver high-quality care across a very wide spectrum of illness. Part of this involves looking after patients who require palliative care, an area of clinical practice which has grown considerably over the years.

The primary care setting has considerable advantages. Patients and their families are generally well known, and this long-term involvement will have allowed trust and respect to develop over the years. Many patients wish to remain at home and to be cared for by their family and friends in a familiar environment. The expertise of the team is considerable and can offer much of the relief and care required.

So much for the background, but how have things changed over the years and how will they develop? First, patients now expect to have greater involvement in their illness and to be communicated with effectively. Their own stories are important and must be listened to, as the example in this book illustrates. They need to have control over their own illness if they so wish. They are increasingly aware of the dilemmas that the team face and the ethical questions which may arise with regard to such issues as pain control, euthanasia and the pressures on carers. They are also aware of the wide range of treatments, including complementary therapies, which are available.

This book considers each of these issues and provides a practical series of ways in which the expertise of both the team as a whole and the individual members of the team can be improved. It includes sections on spiritual aspects of palliative care and the issues surrounding ethnicity and bereavement. In particular, it discusses the issues of palliation in non-malignant conditions. This is very important, as there is considerable experience in the palliation of cancer but much less in other conditions. These non-malignant conditions are often much more difficult to deal with, especially in the younger patient.

Finally, with regard to the team as a whole, two further aspects are considered. The first is how the team will work together. This does not just happen of its own accord. It requires careful planning and working through. Teams do experience conflicts and these need to be dealt with. The changing structure of primary care will provide opportunities to think again about how the team can be built and improved. The second aspect relates to the education of each member of the team. The use of personal development plans is considered as one way of providing an educational route to better care. The second method, involving the use of significant event audit or critical incident analysis, is another powerful tool for change. After all, this is what the whole process is about – changing and improving the quality of life of people who need care and compassion, as well as clinical expertise and humanity, from a competent team. It is our responsibility to provide such a team. Our patients and their families deserve it.

Kenneth C Calman
University of Durham
April 2002

Preface

Perhaps one of the more difficult books to write is one about dying, death and bereavement. With the advent of the specialist hospice movement, there is a feeling among some working in the community that those who are dying should be referred to a Macmillan nurse or palliative medicine specialist, as they believe that they themselves may not have the necessary skills. However, most healthcare professionals look after people with cancer and with progressive chronic incurable illnesses (e.g. chronic obstructive pulmonary disease and multiple sclerosis), where principles of palliation are important. A GP with an average list size may have three to five such patients at any one time, so gaining confidence and skills in this area is important.

Terminal care or palliative care?

Prior to the recognition of the speciality of palliative medicine in 1987 by the Royal College of Physicians, the term most generally used was 'terminal care'. However, the word 'terminal' suggests that death is felt to be certain and not too far off, and so has negative connotations. The term 'palliative' has more positive associations, being associated with maintaining quality of life, and it is applicable to the care of anyone who has an incurable life-threatening disease.

Palliative care or palliative medicine?

For a healthcare professional working within the primary healthcare team (PHCT), this distinction is important. Palliative medicine infers a discipline that is practised by specialists, whereas palliative care is the care provided by a multidisciplinary team of doctors, nurses, therapists, social workers, clergy and volunteers. Thus such care involves much more than the science of symptom control.

What is palliative care?

Many definitions exist, but one of the most helpful has been written by the Royal College of General Practitioners and the Association of Palliative Medicine. It is the care of patients with advanced and progressive disease for whom the focus of care is quality of life and in whom the prognosis is limited, but may be a number of years. It includes consideration of the family's needs before and after the patient's death, as well as bereavement and the care of patients who are dying due to cancer and diseases other than cancer.

Why is palliative care difficult?

As an experienced GP and as the years go by, it doesn't get easier, but in fact more difficult, particularly as one realises that one's turn is getting nearer. I could be criticised by specialists for saying that symptom control is the easy bit. It is not easy unless you have the knowledge, but this can be learned. What cannot be learned easily is how to talk with the person who asks 'Am I dying?' or 'What will it be like?', or who says 'I am frightened.' If you immerse yourself in such intimate and personal consultations, it is difficult. Why is this? It is because it reminds you of your own mortality. Freud summarised this dilemma as follows:

> Our own death is indeed unimaginable and whenever we make the attempt to imagine it we can perceive that we really survive as spectators ... at bottom no one believes in his own death, or to put the same thing in another way, in the unconscious every one of us is convinced of his own immortality.[1]

No wonder, then, that it is difficult to talk to someone about dying.

From being to 'un-being'

In a book on palliative care, you have to start somewhere, and this seems an appropriate place. Gavin Maxwell, the author of *Ring of Bright Water*, went to live in a crofter's cottage in the Highlands of Scotland with his otter 'Mij' to escape life in the big city. He later developed terminal cancer, and he describes the most difficult aspect of this as the 'private and solitary moment of un-being' – the realisation that soon he would no longer exist. Recognising this situation with regard to a patient and helping them to try to come to terms with this difficult prospect is the essence of good palliative care.

Illness: a threat to our very being

> As soon as we are ill we fear that our illness is unique. We argue with ourselves and rationalize, but a ghost of the fear remains. And it remains for a very good reason. The illness, as an undefined force, is a potential threat to our very being.[2]

Being ill is not easy, and healthcare professionals need to be sensitive to their patients. In addition, they need to be prepared to understand and meet the needs created by the threat of an illness to the 'being' of their patients and also to themselves, when that time comes.

Why do we need to get involved?

Many patients are still dying unnecessarily unprepared and suffering, and this is despite the hospice movement and improved teaching. The process starts as soon as a patient receives the bad news of their impending fate. They need access to you as healthcare professionals whenever necessary. You do not need specialist skills, but the time and willingness to talk, empathy for their unfortunate situation, and the ability to explain what treatments such as radiotherapy and chemotherapy involve. This is also something that involves the whole team, and the district nurse should be made aware of such patients as early as possible. As the illness progresses and your relationship of trust develops, review should be regular and organised, whether at the surgery or at the patient's home. In this way crises can be anticipated and unnecessary hospital admissions prevented.

The need to empathise and become involved

In a personal view,[3] a doctor with testicular cancer has described the need to become involved and to empathise. He wrote:

> An analogy to living with cancer is solitary confinement: once inside the prison cell you are trapped; you can walk around, examine the furniture, scrutinise the walls until you know every crack in the plaster, and look out the window; sometimes the door will open and fresh air will enter; yet it is impossible to step over the line dividing the cell from the corridor. The most useful people and the best doctors are those prepared to come inside the cell, sit down, and spend some time with you. Doctors often forget that they are also human.[3]

How many of us would give our home telephone number to a terminally ill patient and their family in such a situation?

'To live until they die'

These are the words of Dame Cicely Saunders, founder of St Christopher's Hospice in London and perhaps, too, of the hospice movement itself. These words emphasise how our role involves enabling the patient to carry on living in this situation.

Symptom control

A GP's role is to enable someone who has an incurable disease to carry on living, where appropriate providing medication to ensure relief of symptoms such as pain, and maintaining their quality of life until they die. There are common symptoms of which those working in the community should be aware, and they should be able to treat these symptoms without referral to a specialist. The four most important symptoms are pain, nausea (with or without vomiting), constipation and fatigue.

Pain control

It is important to overcome the notion that there is an upper limit to the dose of opiate analgesics or a risk of addiction.

Communication, symptom control and morphine

Many treatments are available for symptom relief, especially relief of pain, so there is no excuse for any dying patient being in pain. Skills in symptom control are needed, and it is necessary to overcome the taboo concepts associated with the use of morphine and the false notions that in a dying patient there is a ceiling dose or potential for addiction. The task of communication is important, not least for explaining the need for opiates such as morphine when the time comes, and its implication as perceived by many that this is the end. Paul Egermayer, a doctor who was in this situation himself, wrote a poignant letter to the *New Zealand Medical Journal* last year, and sadly his obituary appeared adjacent to it.

> When to the sometimes bleak prospect of death, which waits us all, is added pain, anguish may result .... To you I send a message of hope. A testimonial to the wonder of MORPHINE and a personal tribute, from someone who is usually very cynical, to that most marvellous product of twentieth-century medicine, PALLIATIVE CARE. It really does work.[4]

This book as a textbook

This book is not intended to be a comprehensive text of palliative medicine, but rather a description of the pertinent issues that constitute primary palliative care. This is important, as the literature reports how the majority of the population, if they have to die, would prefer to die in their own homes rather than in an institution.[5] Yet the opposite happens, with the majority of people dying in hospitals and about one-third dying in the community. The answer is not for everyone to be referred to specialist hospices. The latter are few in number and they are there to act as a catalyst for education and research. In addition, they have a vital role in complicated palliative care scenarios (e.g. where symptom control is not being achieved) by providing advice, specialist day or inpatient care and respite care.

Chapter contributors

The areas of primary palliative care that have been selected for inclusion in this book are relevant to the aim of enabling members of the PHCT to manage dying patients at home where appropriate. The majority of the authors are members of the Centre for Primary Health Care Studies at the University of Warwick, which is also the academic base of three specialists in palliative medicine. We aim to launch a locally and nationally recognised centre (Warwick Palliative Care) in the West Midlands that consists of a partnership between clinical practice, multidisciplinary education in specialist and primary palliative care and research to enhance service delivery and patient care. In addition, we aim to lead palliative care teaching in the new Leicester–Warwick Medical School (LWMS), so that doctors of the future will be better equipped to provide palliative care.

We hope that you will find the book interesting and relevant, and that it will achieve its overall aim of improving care of the dying.

Rodger Charlton
April 2002

References

1 Freud S (1915) Thoughts for the times on war and death. In: *Collected Papers, Volume IV*. Basic Books, New York (collection published in 1959).
2 Berger J and Mohr J (1997) *A Fortunate Man: the story of a country doctor*. Vintage Books, New York.
3 Moreland C (1982) Disabilities and how to live with them: teratoma of the testis. *Lancet.* **i**: 203–5.
4 Egermayer P (2001) A message of hope to those in painful expectation of death (letter). *NZ Med J.* **114**: 367.
5 Charlton R (1991) Attitudes towards care of the dying: a questionnaire survey of general practice attenders. *Fam Pract.* **8**: 356–9.

About the editor

Rodger Charlton BA, MB ChB, MPhil, MD, FRCGP, FRNZCGP, DFFP

Rodger Charlton qualified from Birmingham University. During vocational training in Nottingham he completed an MPhil thesis on medical ethics, entitled 'Medical ethics in terminal care with particular attention to patients dying from leukaemia'. Shortly afterwards he became a GP principal in Derby and a part-time lecturer in general practice at Nottingham University. He was a visiting fellow at the Department of General Practice, University of Otago Medical School, New Zealand in 1991–92, researching into the perceived needs of undergraduates in palliative medicine education. This formed the basis of his MD thesis.

In 1994 he was appointed senior lecturer in primary healthcare at the Postgraduate School of Medicine, Keele University, and in 1995 he took over a single-handed general practice in Hampton-in-Arden, close to the Warwickshire border. In 1996 he was appointed as a research fellow at the NHS Executive GP Unit, where he was involved in creating a palliative care training programme for GP registrars. In 1997 he became a GP trainer and in 1998 he became editor of the Royal College of General Practitioners (RCGP) *Members' Reference Book* (*MRB*) for two years. He is now editor of RCGP publications (excluding the journal and *MRB*).

His research interests and published papers are in the fields of palliative care, bereavement and meningococcal disease, but there is a strong focus on research in education and professional development in primary care. In September 2000 he was appointed senior lecturer in continuing professional development at Warwick University. In April 2001 he received the John Fry Award from the Royal College of General Practitioners, for a GP who has promoted the discipline of general practice through research and publishing as a practising GP.

About the contributors

Mandy Barnett BSc, MB BS, MD, MRCGP, DMRT
Mandy Barnett is Macmillan Consultant in Palliative Medicine at Walsgrave Hospitals NHS Trust, and she joined the University of Warwick in October 1996. She provides clinical leadership to the Coventry Macmillan Palliative Care Team, and consultant supervision to Myton Hamlet Hospice in Warwick. She graduated from University College Hospital, London, and completed her postgraduate training in London and Bristol. At Bristol University she worked on aspects of doctor–patient communication, the effects of medical education on communication skills, and the psychological status of patients with advanced cancer.

Barry Clark BSc, PhD, MA, MSc
Barry Clark trained initially as an animal nutritionist, and was then ordained for the ministry. He obtained his BSc at Newcastle University and then gained a PhD in tryptophan metabolism. He subsequently studied theology at Oxford for his MA, and later medical ethics at Birmingham University for his MSc. He has been a full-time chaplain at Selly Oak Hospital, Birmingham, for nine years and he specialises in medical ethics. He is Chairman of the Palliative Care Development Group at the University Hospital Birmingham NHS Trust.

Tim Deegan MB BS, DCH, DRCOG
After completing general practice training in Hereford in 1997, Tim Deegan worked as a locum for two years before joining the staff at Myton Hamlet Hospice, Warwick. He is currently working as a general practitioner, having just completed a year as an academic GP registrar at the Centre for Primary Health Care Studies, University of Warwick.

Joanne Fisher BSc, PhD
After completing her BSc and PhD at Warwick University in the Department of Psychology, Joanne Fisher joined the Centre for Primary Health Care Studies, University of Warwick, in October 2000 as a Research Fellow to work on the *Breaking Bad News* project to implement and evaluate innovative training methods for hospital consultants. She is also a part-time lecturer at Coventry University.

Wolfram Jatsch MRCGP, DFFP, DTM&H
Wolfram Jatsch went to medical school in Milan and qualified in Munich in 1994. He undertook all of his hospital and GP training in the UK, and recently completed a post as an academic GP registrar in the Centre for Primary Health Care Studies, University of Warwick. He is currently working as a general practitioner, and his main research interest is in the information needs of patients with prostate cancer.

Karen Mills BSc
After graduating from Imperial College, University of London, with a degree in life sciences, Karen Mills worked as a sub-editor for the *British Journal of General Practice*. She then spent 12 years carrying out research in general practice at the Department of General Practice, Queen's University, Belfast, after which she worked for Warwickshire Health Authority for seven years, first as manager of the Medical Audit Advisory Group and then as Clinical Governance Manager. During this time she maintained her research interest via her role as an Associate Fellow at Warwick University. She is currently working as a Health Care Consultant for Pfizer, where her role includes the development of joint projects with the NHS to support implementation of the National Service Frameworks.

Dan Munday MB BS, FFARCSI, DRCOG, MRCGP, Dip.Pall.Med.
After qualifying in 1982, and completing general professional training in anaesthesia, Dan Munday spent three years (1988–91) in Nepal, where he was responsible for anaesthetic service development and training in rural Nepali hospitals. On returning to the UK, he entered general practice, working as a GP principal in Aberdeen, where he was involved in undergraduate medical education at the University of Aberdeen. He has just completed specialist registrar training in palliative medicine, and is a visiting senior lecturer at the Centre for Primary Health Care Studies, University of Warwick. He has a research interest in the interface between primary and secondary palliative care, including the provision of 'out-of-hours' care for terminally ill patients and the application of complexity theory to the field of palliative care.

Ina Murphy
Ina Murphy is a retired teacher who has personally been on the cancer journey. She uses her skills and experience in talking to groups about her illness and the role of healthcare professionals in caring for the terminally ill. She provides a unique insight into the impact of cancer as a life-threatening disease on a person's life.

Jo Piercy MB ChB, MRCP, MRCGP
Prior to her general practice training, Jo Piercy worked as a specialist registrar in haematology for 18 months. This gave her an insight into the challenges that are faced by those who manage dying patients and their families. She entered general practice after a 12-month post as an aademic GP registrar at the Centre for Primary Health Care Studies, University of Warwick. She has just been appointed as a lecturer in general practice at Birmingham University.

Carole Anne Tallon BSc, MB ChB, MRCGP, DFFP
After studying biological sciences and psychology at Leicester University, Carole Anne Tallon studied medicine at the same university. She then undertook several years of varied Senior House Officer posts and worked in Australia as a rural GP locum in 1995. She then returned to England to complete general practice training, and is now completing specialist training in palliative medicine. Her special interests include communication, teaching, geriatric medicine and the links between primary and secondary palliative care.

Derek Willis MB ChB (Hons), MRCP
After training as a physician in Birmingham and gaining his MRCP in 1996, Derek Willis trained in palliative medicine. He is now a full-time GP and hospital practitioner in palliative medicine at University Hospital, Birmingham. His main research interest is medical ethics, and he is an honorary clinical lecturer in the Department of Primary Care, University of Birmingham.

John Wilmot MB ChB, FRCGP
After graduating from Birmingham University and undertaking vocational training in the city, John Wilmot joined a large group teaching practice in Leamington Spa. He has been a trainer and a vocational training course organiser, and is currently a co-ordinating tutor for academic registrars based at Warwick University. He helped to establish the multidisciplinary Diploma/Masters course in primary care management at the University of Warwick, where he has been a senior lecturer since 1984. His research interests include continuing professional development and quality improvement.

Alexandra Withnall BA, MA, PhD
After working as a Staff Tutor in the Department of Continuing Education at Lancaster University, Alexandra Withnall taught in the School of Postgraduate Medicine at Keele University. Until recently she was a lecturer within the Leicester–Warwick Medical School, and she is now the Director of Continuing Professional Development in the Centre for Primary Health Care Studies, University of Warwick. Her research has focused on aspects of social gerontology and on the development of lifelong learning, as well as her current interest in aspects of bereavement. At present, she is Chair of the Association for Education and Ageing.

CHAPTER 1

The development of palliative care within primary care

Mandy Barnett

Introduction

In this introductory chapter the historical context of care of the dying is reviewed, as well as the evolution of terminal care into the modern field of palliative care. Some of the services available to people with palliative care needs in the community, and the interface between primary care and specialist palliative care, will be described in the context of ongoing changes in demography and organisation of the health service in the UK today.

Historical context

The modern hospice movement in the UK is largely considered to date from the opening of St Christopher's Hospice in 1967. However, the original concept of a hospice as a place of rest for weary travellers dates back many hundreds of years to a time when religious institutions welcomed and tended pilgrims. This gradually evolved into care of the sick and dying. Associated as they were with Catholic organisations, hospices disappeared during the Reformation. The first 'modern' hospice was founded in France in 1842. In the UK, three Protestant Homes of Rest were founded in the late 1800s, while St Joseph's Hospice, which opened in London in 1905, offered care for the dying through its order of nursing sisters.[1]

Role of the doctor

Care of the dying was not considered to be the province of the physician until the nineteenth century.[2] Since then, the medical profession has increasingly accepted responsibility for end-of-life care, but not without difficulty. Over the last 50 years there has been increasing reliance on technical advances, together with devaluation of the more subtle concept of doctor as healer. Alongside this, improvements in public health medicine have increased life expectancy in the Western world from 50 years at the beginning of the twentieth century[3] to 80 years in 2001. However, although death may be postponed, it remains inevitable. Yet ironically, as our society becomes more open about sexual and emotional issues, death has retreated to become a taboo area. In the hospital setting, death may be seen as a failure for which doctors are ill prepared by their training. As Balfour Mount pointed out: 'when medical technology doesn't know what to do, the quality and quantity of care falls away. How can we justify that?'[4]

Hospice movement

It was the increasing sense of depersonalisation in the acute hospital setting which provoked Dame Cicely Saunders, the founder of St Christopher's Hospice, to break away and develop a modern hospice where care of the dying individual would entail total care.

The first new charitably funded hospices concentrated on offering inpatient services for people who would otherwise have died in acute hospital wards. However, they soon expanded their horizons to develop home-care teams, day centres, hospice at home, bereavement support and specialist services such as lymphoedema clinics. Gradually, too, the NHS began to recognise the need for such services and to take on increasing responsibility for funding. This led to the setting up of hospital support teams and the building of the first entirely NHS hospices in the 1970s. At that time, patients were usually those with a prognosis of days or weeks, and hospice care was therefore known as terminal care. The majority of patients had cancer, although some hospices had a more open policy, catering for patients with progressive neurological conditions, and more recently those with AIDS.

Terminal care or palliative care?

The change in terminology from terminal care to palliative care reflected the growing perception that the palliative care approach would benefit all of those living with a terminal or life-limiting disease, and not just those in the final stages. Gradually, as more hospices developed and more professionals worked in them, the concept of a specialist multidisciplinary field of palliative care evolved. For doctors, this culminated in the recognition of palliative medicine as a specialty by the Royal College of Physicians in 1987, which led to the development of a career path and training programme. Similarly, for other healthcare professionals there are now a variety of postgraduate training programmes and higher degrees in palliative care. Today, palliative care is viewed as an integral part of mainstream healthcare.

What is palliative care? Terms of reference

Terminal care is a fairly self-explanatory concept. Palliative care is a more nebulous term arising from the classical *'pallium'* (Latin for cloak or cover). The modern definition in the *Oxford Dictionary* is a little more helpful: 'Palliate: to mitigate, alleviate, give temporary relief'.

A more comprehensive healthcare definition has been provided by the World Health Organization:

> The active total care of patients whose disease is not responsive to curative treatment. Control of pain, of other symptoms and of psychological, social and spiritual problems is paramount. The goal of palliative care is achievement of the best quality of life for patients and their families. ... Palliative care ... offers a support system to help patients live as actively as possible until death ... offers a support system to help the family cope during the patient's illness and in their own bereavement.[5]

Palliative care in primary care
Needs and service provision

While hospital specialists have struggled with care of the dying, the concept of holistic care for people at all life stages forms a fundamental principle of primary care. For most people with a terminal illness, their aim is to live in their own homes, to be cared for physically, to have distressing symptoms alleviated as far as is possible, and to be treated and respected as autonomous individuals. To enable these needs to be met, there is a wide range of services that may be accessed by patients and their families (*see* Box 1.1).

Box 1.1   Services available to palliative care patients in the primary care setting (comprehensive but not exhaustive)

Primary care team:
  GP district nurse
  Marie Curie nurses
  Social Services (e.g. home-care support)
  Community/cottage hospitals
  Nursing homes – for respite or long-term care
  Other generic services: community pharmacists, physiotherapists, podiatrists, etc.)

Specialist services:
  Macmillan (or equivalent) specialist community nurses with or without consultant in palliative medicine
  Hospice at Home
  Hospice/palliative care day centres

Living and dying at home – the impact of social and organisational change on primary and palliative care

Palliative care has always been a feature of primary care. Most people spend 90% of their last year in the community, and the majority would also prefer to die at home.[6,7] The paradox is that the more 'advanced' a society becomes, the less likely it is that this final wish will be fulfilled. There are two aspects to the problem, namely symptom control and home-care support.

Symptom control in primary care

Good symptom control has two essential ingredients, namely good communication (with patients and carers and between healthcare professionals) and a problem-based assessment of the possible therapeutic options. This requires a detailed knowledge of both pharmacological and non-pharmacological interventions. A general practitioner who is looking after an average of five to ten patients per year with palliative care needs is unlikely to be able to keep up with either new pharmacological developments or the benefits of treatments such as palliative radiotherapy or chemotherapy.[8]

Surveys in the 1980s certainly found that many general practitioners (32%) struggled with pain control.[9] Although many GPs receive training in symptom control during their registrar year,[10] this is limited, and a survey of new GP principals found that they were uncertain about basic principles with regard to opioid prescription.[11] Furthermore, GPs may not update their knowledge subsequently. Among GPs who were referring to a hospice inpatient unit, 37% had not attended any educational event pertinent to palliative care during the past 3 years. Among patients referred by this group, a common symptom was constipation secondary to inadequate prescribing of aperients alongside opiates.[12] This was corroborated by a study of patients' relatives, which indicated comparatively fewer instances of poor pain control (15%), but still significant problems with other symptoms.[13]

Social and nursing care: a demographic time-bomb

It is well recognised that in Western society the population is ageing, as life expectancy increases and the birth rate decreases. Many older people live healthier, more independent lives than previous generations. However, for those whose health deteriorates, there is less informal support available in the community and more reliance on professional carers than ever before. A number of social and demographic factors contribute to this situation, including the following.

1   *Social mobility and the demise of the extended family.* Accelerating changes in employment patterns have led to families becoming more widely scattered. Relatives often live too far away to contribute practical care. Conversely, as communities become more transient, people receive less contact and support from neighbours.

2   *Ageing population.* Children of the elderly are becoming fewer and are themselves older.

3   *Time to care.* Changing work patterns, increasing prevalence and costs of home ownership and increasing divorce rates mean that many would-be carers rely on dual incomes, or are lone parents (often isolated), and thus have less time to care for dependent relatives.

4   *Changes in social attitudes.* Death at any age has become an increasingly remote event, with dying being a medical rather than a social process. Many young people have had little first-hand experience of death, and feel inadequately prepared to cope with the emotional and physical needs of someone with a life-limiting condition.

Patients and relatives have increasingly high expectations of professional care. Equally, however, both relatives and professionals are aware of the limitations of the services available. In one large survey, inadequacies in the level of home help and district nursing provision were perceived both to affect care and to discourage relatives from caring for a dying person.[14]

This reinforces the results of a survey of the place of death of cancer patients.[15] This survey found that hospital or hospice admission was most commonly due to problems in providing care. In 22% of cases there was no lay carer, while in 45% of cases the lay carer became unable to continue to provide care.

The changing role of the general practitioner

It has been argued that care of a hospice type can be provided by any general practitioner who is interested in care of the dying.[16] The key factors include utilising a team approach (especially maintaining close communication with nurses), developing skills in symptom control, being prepared to take the extra time and effort necessary to foresee and alleviate potential problems, and communicating with the patient and his or her family.

The majority of general practitioners still regard the care of patients with palliative care needs as an inherent and important part of their role.[17]

However, this must be squared with radical changes in the organisation of primary care. The majority of general practitioners now work in multi-partner practices, with fewer practices operating personal lists. Consequently, there is greater flexibility but potentially less continuity for patients. Routine daytime visiting has considerably decreased, while increasing public demand for a 24-hour rather than emergency service has led to major changes in the delivery of out-of-hours care which, except for the most isolated rural practices, is now largely devolved to co-operatives or deputising services.

This can be problematic in palliative care. A recent survey of GPs in rural and inner-city areas found that although 75% still personally provided palliative care out of hours, 23% handed over all care to out-of-hours organisations.[18] There is evidence that information about terminally ill patients is not reliably transferred to co-operatives operating out-of-hours cover, resulting in poor continuity of care.[19]

The role of GP facilitators in palliative care

These innovative posts were set up and funded by Macmillan Cancer Relief in the 1990s to help to develop palliative care within primary care (currently there are about 60 posts). GP facilitators are practising general practitioners with an interest in palliative medicine. Their remit is wide and varies from one region to another, but it includes the following:

1   reviewing the current state of local community palliative care
2   exploring the needs of local practitioners and supporting service initiatives
3   offering support and encouraging the development of educational initiatives
4   facilitating working relationships with specialist services (e.g. improving awareness of out-of-hours advisory services).

They may also have an advisory role at an organisational level, helping to define palliative care service needs. This has become particularly relevant to the development of primary care trusts (PCTs) and the need for cancer accreditation in primary care.

Continuity of care, teamwork and the role of district nurses

Teamwork is essential for the effective delivery of palliative care in any setting. Frequently the district nurse is the palliative care linchpin of the primary care team. Prompt referral to district nurses is extremely important for assessment of needs, family support and continuity of care. Unfortunately, although they appreciate the role of the district nurse, general practitioners may not always refer patients early enough, possibly reflecting their awareness of the fact that the service is over-stretched.[20]

Teamwork can be improved by implementing a multidisciplinary approach to palliative care within the primary care team. This was demonstrated in Newcastle by a project that provided facilitators to set up auditable guidelines for practices. This improved the understanding of different professional roles, as well as contributing a multidisciplinary perspective to the guidelines themselves.[21]

Out of hours, good teamwork may make the difference between patients remaining at home and being admitted to hospital. Doctor–doctor communication can be enhanced if co-operatives develop protocols for handing over information about terminally ill patients, leading to more consistent advice and reducing the likelihood of emergency call-outs and inappropriate admissions.

Nursing support is particularly relevant to families, both for reassurance and to alleviate the physical burden of caring. Here, manpower as well as communication is an issue. Provision of out-of-hours district nursing and night nursing services is inconsistent across the country, which may exacerbate the problem of otherwise unnecessary admissions to hospital.[17,22]

Marie Curie nurses

This charitably funded service provides practical hands-on nursing care in patients' homes, using trained nurses who have received additional induction and in-service training to enable them to meet palliative care needs. They provide both daytime and out-of-hours care, and they are an invaluable resource to district nursing services. As with all palliative care services, there are not enough to go round, and although flexible, they do not provide an emergency service. However, where Marie Curie services are available there is evidence that they facilitate patients remaining at home.[23]

Role of specialist palliative care services in primary care

Specialist palliative care services are involved with 50% or more of all patients who are terminally ill with cancer in the UK. They are also involved with an increasing proportion of patients at earlier stages in their illness, where there are difficult symptoms, psychological needs or complex social issues. They may extend their role to patients with other diagnoses – a role that is expanding although much less consistent.

Services range from multi-bedded academic inpatient units to stand-alone day centres.

Whatever their make-up, the common aims of specialist services are as follows:

- to improve the quality of life of patients and their families
- to support professionals involved in direct care
- to ascertain and respond to the educational needs of healthcare professionals
- to promote and develop audit and research in areas relating to palliative care.

This chapter will focus on the relationship between these services and primary care, and will only briefly describe the services themselves (hospital teams are omitted for this reason, although some hospital teams are integrated into the community and can be considered in this context).

Specialist palliative care inpatient units

The size and shape of inpatient units vary enormously across the UK, with many voluntary hospices having been built and funded as a result of local public appeal.

The minimum number of beds considered to be economically viable is about 14, although larger facilities have become increasingly popular. Admission is generally considered for one of the following requirements:

- symptom control (including psychological needs)
- terminal care
- assessment and rehabilitation
- respite (for patient and/or family).

Day hospice/palliative care day centre

Day hospices offer a variety of services to home-based patients, and help to provide a non-threatening introduction to palliative care services. Most of them operate daily during the week, providing a social programme, complementary therapies, bathing and hairdressing facilities. They may also offer access to physiotherapy, occupational therapy and medical review, and some of them offer specialist lymphoedema clinics. As the pressure on inpatient units grows, some centres are now also providing day-case facilities for supportive procedures such as blood transfusion and bisphosphonate infusion for pain control.

Hospice at Home

The term *Hospice at Home* covers a multitude of service models, most of which have been developed according to local need, shaped by the availability of other services and financial or manpower constraints. They may involve a complete 24-hour nursing outreach service,[1.1] or provide a co-ordinating role and specialist support to ensure continuity of care with existing community services.

Specialist palliative care community teams

Specialist community teams may be entirely community based, or linked to independent or NHS hospices or hospital services (including those integrated with hospital support teams). Organisation and membership of the team vary, but it usually consists of specialist nurses and consultant physicians plus administrative support. Other professionals (e.g. social worker) may be integral or accessed as needed.

[1.1] A 24-hour service is provided by the Iain Rennie Hospice at Home model, a service based in Hertfordshire, described in National Council for Hospice and Specialist Palliative Care Services Paper 15, *Promoting Partnership: Planning and Managing Community Palliative Care*, published in 1998.

Specialist palliative care/primary care interface

There are two major points of interface between specialist palliative care and primary care services:

1   home care
2   admission to specialist inpatient beds.

Home care

At its best, involvement of the palliative care team can provide both professionals and the patient with support, leading to improved symptom control, reduced anxiety and improved co-ordination of care. Most teams work in an advisory capacity. However, the interface between specialists and members of the primary care team caring for a patient at home is not always clearly defined. General practitioners and district nurses can sometimes feel that their role is being usurped, although usually specialist input is perceived as helpful.[24] Interestingly, community specialist nurse input is more likely to be appreciated by district nurses than by general practitioners, and is likely to be viewed more negatively by those who have had least contact with the service.[20]

It is important for both patients and professionals that the specialist role is understood and put to optimal use by the primary care team. Equally, it is important for specialists and those involved in service development to understand the primary care view of what is needed. This requires communication and negotiation.

The most important message from GPs has been the need for clear communication with the specialist team, but a more global concern relates to input for patients with non-malignant disease, and improved out-of-hours access.[25] Simple practical measures can be useful (e.g. in our local community, a survey of general practitioners led to the review of palliative care team documentation and the creation of a database to record GPs' communication preferences).[1.2]

Admission to specialist inpatient beds

One of the failings of specialist palliative care cited by GPs and district nurses is the lack of access to beds, both in the daytime and out of hours. It is becoming increasingly difficult to obtain admission for an individual who is simply dying.

Equally, for palliative care units, a constant problem is that of balancing the needs of patients in the unit with those on the waiting-list. To meet the demand, most specialist units operate a policy of short-stay admissions (averaging 14 days), and will not admit patients with longer-term needs unless there are both current specialist needs and clear identification of an onward (e.g. nursing home) placement. This policy aims to avoid distressing patients by multiple moves, but it potentially

---

[1.2] Reddall C (1999) *Coventry Macmillan Palliative Care Team.* Unpublished paper.

discriminates against those who are dependent but not yet dying.[26] The other inpatient options that exist are listed below.

GP-led hospices

Before the existence of specialist palliative care, many voluntary sector hospices were staffed by general practitioners with an interest in palliative care. With the advent of specialist palliative medicine, some of these became full-time consultants, while others elected to remain as GPs. This led to the division of independent hospices into specialist and generic palliative care units. GP-led services are unable to provide training for junior doctors, and may be limited in implementing innovations in practice, but they provide consistent patient care and thus remain a valuable resource.

Community hospitals

In rural settings, community hospitals have an important role, enabling patients to be cared for nearer to home, in a more intimate, less 'high-tech' environment, with continuity provided by their own GPs. However, there has been little evaluation of the role of community hospitals in the provision of palliative care. Access to a community hospital has been shown to reduce the number of deaths occurring in the specialist cancer unit.[27] However, comparison of care provided by community hospitals and specialist hospices has invoked some criticism of the community hospitals with regard to communication, bereavement support and nurse staffing levels.[28] While staffing levels may not always be easily addressed, other issues can be resolved through education.

Private nursing homes

With the closure of long-term NHS beds, the care of dependent frail people has increasingly fallen to lay carers or to private nursing homes. This has led to a very real shortfall in the availability of medium-term beds for patients with palliative care needs.

Nursing homes with palliative care beds may offer a middle ground. They aim to provide a permanent home for patients who are deteriorating at a slower rate, and who require levels of nursing care that are unavailable to them at home, but whose symptoms are stable or easily controlled. To take on this function, such nursing homes must provide levels of trained staff and medical cover in accordance with health authority requirements, and access to specialist advice must still be available.

However, for patients and their families to accept a nursing-home place as a viable alternative to a hospice, they must be confident that the levels of nursing care provided are adequate, and that the knowledge of symptom control measures is appropriate to the needs of dying patients. Studies of this area indicate a considerable need for education before these standards can be met.[29,30] However, education projects aimed at nursing-home staff do feature as a new major funding initiative resulting from the NHS Cancer Plan proposed by the Department of Health. Thus it is hoped that this option will prove increasingly acceptable to patients and their families.

Palliative care for non-cancer diagnoses

Much of the emphasis of specialist palliative care has been on cancer care. This reflects both the specific physical and emotional challenges associated with cancer, and a historical need to establish expertise in one disease area, to encourage the development of a research base and to increase the visibility and credibility of healthcare professionals. In addition, much of the funding originates from the voluntary sector, in particular Macmillan Cancer Relief.[1.3] Macmillan has established an increasingly important profile in funding the development of specialist posts and in building hospices. Although not proscriptive, for most consumers of these services and their healthcare professionals, Macmillan is synonymous with cancer.

However, while the needs of cancer patients have not diminished, there is increasing recognition that patients with other conditions (e.g. cardiac failure) suffer from equally distressing symptoms, and face similar emotional and social difficulties.[31] At present, though, access to specialist palliative care advice is more limited for these groups, and they are less likely to be referred by their GPs.[32] From the perspective of specialist palliative care teams, there may be educational and manpower issues that limit present capacity to offer a wider service,[33] although services that currently offer open access perceive their skills to be transferable to non-cancer diagnoses.[34] However, this situation can and must be addressed by training programmes and by funding bodies. It is a sad reflection of affairs when families comment that patients are 'lucky' to have had cancer. It is no more acceptable for people to face a diagnostic lottery for palliative care than it is to have a postcode lottery for treatment.

Summary

Palliative care has come a long way, but it occupies a unique position as a multidisciplinary specialty which remains inextricably linked with primary care, both in its diversity of settings and in its holistic view of patients and their families. One of the challenges with regard to integrating modern-day palliative and primary care is to recognise the resources that each brings to the care of the

---

[1.3] This charitable organisation (originally named the Society for the Prevention and Relief of Cancer) was founded by a young man called Douglas Macmillan, following the harrowing death of his father from cancer in 1911. Its aim was to inform professionals and the public about cancer, and it became increasingly involved with providing practical help to sufferers and their families. In 1924, it distributed £11 in grants to patients; this reached £1.5 million in 1982 and increased exponentially to £5.1 million in 1999. By the end of the 1960s, the charity funded the building of three hospices; the first Macmillan nurse posts were established in 1975, and this figure had climbed to 2000 by the end of the year 2000 (Macmillan website: http://www.macmillan.org.uk).

individual, and to use those resources to maximum effect. Current specialist manpower and bed provision cannot meet the face-to-face needs of all individual patients. However, there is scope to meet those needs if we focus on improving communication, making relevant education available for different professional groups, and providing accessible advisory support to lay carers and professionals both at home and in other community settings.

All members of the primary healthcare team value aspects of specialist palliative care. In particular, the ability to admit patients urgently is seen both as a need in itself and, conversely, as a means of keeping people in their own homes for longer. For patients at home, access to domiciliary specialist medical advice, specialist nursing input and night-time Marie Curie services are all seen as valuable services that require expansion. Above all, the impact of specialist palliative care on cancer care has served to highlight the need for the same facilities to be made available to all patients, whatever their diagnosis.

References

1 Saunders C (1996) Foreword, In: D Doyle, GWC Hanks and N MacDonald (eds) *Oxford Textbook of Palliative Medicine*. Oxford University Press, Oxford.

2 Bodemer CW (1979) Physicians and the dying: a historical sketch. *J Fam Pract.* **9**: 827–32.

3 Fry J (1993) *General Practice: the facts*. Radcliffe Medical Press, Oxford.

4 Hamilton J (1995) Dr Balfour Mount and the cruel irony of our care for the dying. *Can Med Assoc J.* **153**: 334-6.

5 World Health Organization (1990) *Cancer Pain Relief and Palliative Care*. Technical Report Series 804. World Health Organization, Geneva.

6 Townsend J, Frank A, Fermont D, Dyer S, Karren O and Walgrove A (1990) Terminal cancer and patients' preference for a place of death: a prospective study. *BMJ.* **301**: 415–17.

7 Charlton RC (1991) Attitudes towards care of the dying: a questionnaire survey of general practice attenders. *Fam Pract.* **8**: 356–9.

8 Barnes EA, Hanson J, Neumann CM, Nekolaichuk CL and Bruera E (2000) Communication between primary care physicians and radiation oncologists regarding patients with cancer treated with palliative radiotherapy. *J Clin Oncol.* **18**: 2902–7.

9 Haines A and Booroff A (1986) Terminal care at home: perspective from general practice. *BMJ.* **292**: 1051–3.

10 Barclay S, Todd C, Grande G and Lipscombe J (1997) How common is medical training in palliative care? A postal survey of general practitioners. *Br J Gen Pract.* **47**: 800–4.

11 Lloyd-Williams M and Lloyd-Williams F (1996) Palliative care teaching and today's general practitioners – is it adequate? *Eur J Cancer Care.* **5**: 242–5.

12 Seamark DA, Lawrence C and Gilbert J (1996) Characteristics of referrals to an inpatient hospice and a survey of general practitioner perceptions of palliative care. *J R Soc Med.* **89**: 79–84.

13 Millar DG, Carroll D, Grimshaw J and Watt B (1998) Palliative care at home: an audit of cancer deaths in Grampian region. *Br J Gen Pract.* **48**: 1299–302.

14 Cartwright A (1991) Balance of care for the dying between hospitals and the community: perceptions of general practitioners, hospital consultants, community nurses and relatives. *Br J Gen Pract.* **41**: 271–4.

15 Herd EB (1990) Terminal care in a semi-rural area. *Br J Gen Pract.* **40**: 248–51.

16 MacAdam DB (1983) Care of the dying. Relevance of the hospice concept to general practice. *Austr Fam Physician.* **12**: 249–50.

17 Pugh EMG (1996) An investigation of general practitioner referrals to palliative care services. *Palliative Med.* **10**: 251–7.

18 Shipman C, Addington-Hall J, Barclay S *et al.* (2000) Providing palliative care in primary care: how satisfied are GPs and district nurses with current out-of-hours arrangements? *Br J Gen Pract.* **50**: 477–8.

19 Barclay S, Rogers M and Todd C (1997) Communication between GPs and co-operatives is poor for terminally ill patients. *BMJ.* **315**: 1235–6.

20 Cartwright A (1991) The relationship between general practitioners, hospital consultants and community nurses when caring for people in the last year of their lives. *Fam Pract.* **8**: 350–5.

21 Robinson L and Stacy R (1994) Palliative care in the community: setting practice guidelines for primary care teams. *Br J Gen Pract.* **44**: 461–4.

22 Jones Elwyn G and Stott N (1994) Avoidable referrals? Analysis of 170 consecutive referrals to secondary care. *BMJ.* **309**: 576–8.

23 Higginson IJ and Wilkinson S (2000) Do Marie Curie nurses enable more patients with advanced cancer to remain and die at home in the UK? *Palliative Med.* **14**: 246.

24 Robbins MA, Jackson P and Prentice A (1996) Statutory and voluntary sector palliative care in the community setting: National Health Service professionals' perceptions of the interface. *Eur J Cancer Care.* **5**: 96–102.

25 Higginson I (1999) Palliative care services in the community: what do family doctors want? *J Palliative Care.* **15**: 21–5.

26 Addington-Hall J, Altmann D and McCarthy M (1998) Which terminally ill cancer patients receive hospice inpatient care? *Soc Sci Med.* **46**: 1011–16.

27 Thorne CP, Seamark DA, Lawrence C and Gray DJ (1994) The influence of general practitioner community hospitals on the place of death of cancer patients. *Palliative Med.* **8**: 122–8.

28 Seamark DA, Williams S, Hall M, Lawrence CJ and Gilbert J (1998) Dying from cancer in community hospitals or a hospice: closest lay carer's perceptions. *Br J Gen Pract.* **48**: 1317–21.

29 Gibbs G (1995) Nurses in private nursing homes: a study of their knowledge and attitudes to pain management in palliative care. *Palliative Med.* **9**: 245–53.

30 Sidell M, Katz J and Komaromy C (1998) *Death and Dying in Residential and Nursing Homes for Older People: examining the case for palliative care.* Open University Press, Buckingham.

31 Addington-Hall JM, Fakhoury W and McCarthy M (1998) Specialist palliative care in non-malignant disease. *Palliative Med.* **12**: 417–27.

32 Kurti LG and O'Dowd TC (1995) Dying of non-malignant disease in general practice. *J Palliative Care.* **11**: 25–31.

33 Addington-Hall J (1998) *Reaching Out: specialist palliative care for adults with non-malignant diseases.* Occasional Paper 14. National Council for Hospice and Specialist Palliative Care Services, London.
34 Kite S, Jones K and Tookman A (1999) Specialist palliative care and patients with non-cancer diagnoses: the experience of a service. *Palliative Med.* **13**: 477–84.

Useful websites

Association for Palliative Medicine; www.palliative-medicine.org
European Association for Palliative Care; http://www.eapcnet.org/home.html
National Hospice Council; www.hospice-spc-council.org.uk/

CHAPTER 2

Clinical governance and palliative care

Dan Munday

The term *clinical governance* first appeared in 1997 in the White Paper entitled *A First-Class Service*.[1] The Government has defined it as:

> A framework through which NHS organisations are accountable for continuously improving the quality of their service and safeguarding high standards of care, by creating an environment in which excellence in clinical care will flourish.[1]

All NHS organisations, including primary care groups (PCGs), primary care trusts (PCTs), health authorities (HAs) and acute hospital trusts (AHTs), are required to take part in clinical governance. Although the term has come into common usage, it has caused much confusion.

What is clinical governance?

The concept of what has become known as clinical governance is not new – certainly most of its features, which are discussed in this chapter, have been central to quality control within primary care for many years. They have featured within primary care quality indicators such as the Quality Practice Award (QPA) and Fellowship By Assessment (FBA) of the Royal College of General Practitioners.

The role of the PCG/PCT

In primary care, either the PCG (which is a subcommittee of a health authority) or the PCT (an independent NHS trust) are the organisations responsible for clinical governance. PCGs/PCTs have been required to establish leadership in clinical governance by establishing either a clinical governance lead practitioner or a subcommittee. They are expected to set up accountability arrangements for primary care practitioners, baseline assessment of activity in primary care and action planning. They are also expected to put in place reporting arrangements to ensure that clinical governance takes place. Practices are not directly involved in clinical governance, but if PCTs are to engage in meaningful governance activity, it needs to be performed largely within practices and with the co-operation of the whole primary care team.

The principles of clinical governance are clearly relevant to practices and will be embraced by many as being a positive tool for practice development. Most practices will find that establishing a 'lead professional' for clinical governance provides a focus for it and enables the practice to ensure that the area is addressed. This lead may be a partner, the practice manager or a practice nurse. Larger partnerships may find that a multidisciplinary clinical governance group rather than a single lead professional is more appropriate. In addition, PCTs should be able to provide practical help for practices through their own clinical governance 'leads' and committees.

Components of clinical governance

The central features of clinical governance are accountability, quality control and improving standards. A multiprofessional approach and acknowledgement of the importance of organisational structures in the delivery of high-quality care are essential for effective clinical governance. Finally, involvement of patients – 'the users of the service' – is encouraged to ensure accountability to the community in addition to accountability to the higher management structures within the NHS (*see* Figure 2.1). The aim is ultimately to protect the public from poor practice as well as to drive services towards the delivery of excellent care.

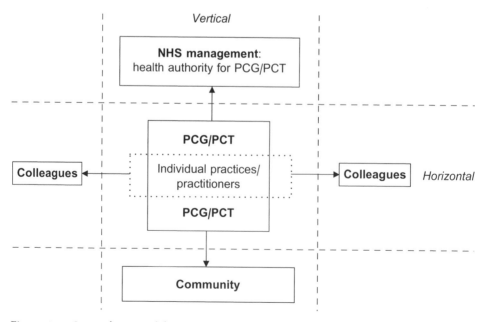

Figure 2.1 Lines of accountability.

Accountability

Healthcare professionals are accountable to their professional registration bodies. In the case of doctors this is the General Medical Council (GMC), and in the case of nurses it is the United Kingdom Central Committee for Nurse Registration (UKCC). The concept of this professional accountability is such that individual practitioners are responsible for their own actions, and they are answerable to their registration body for any failure in their professional standards. Such failure may result in disciplinary action being taken against them. The penalties can vary from following a mandatory retraining programme to removal of registration and consequently the licence to practise.

In addition, within primary care, general practitioner principals are responsible, by way of their contract with health authorities, for fulfilling agreed 'terms of service'. Health authorities may take disciplinary action against general practitioners if they fail to fulfil these terms. The general practitioner is also responsible, on the basis of their contract, for the actions of their employed staff involved in the care of their registered patients. Criticisms of this system include the facts that it is adversarial in nature, it is based on maintaining minimum standards rather than ensuring quality, and it relies on patients or their relatives highlighting failures through complaints.

Professional self-regulation of doctors through the GMC has come under increasing scrutiny in recent years, with accusations – as a result of high-profile cases – that this system fails to protect patients adequately. The adversarial nature of dealing with complaints in primary care has also fostered a notion of professionals 'closing ranks' to protect colleagues from discipline. Aims to redress this problem were introduced before the advent of clinical governance with the introduction of practice-based complaints systems to deal with complaints promptly and with transparency. Ultimately, however, accountability still rested on complaints being made against individual practitioners.

Clinical governance seeks to increase and formalise the accountability of healthcare professionals and NHS organisations by specifically introducing three areas of accountability. These are accountability of individual practitioners for the actions of team colleagues (so-called *horizontal accountability*), accountability of the organisation to NHS management and accountability of the organisation to the community (so-called *vertical accountability*) (*see* Figure 2.1). The accountability of health professionals for each other's practice aims to foster a sense of collective responsibility for clinical practice within the healthcare organisation.

Quality control and improving standards

Primary care teams should be delivering high-quality care for all patients. There are many ways in which quality can be assessed (*see* section on tools of clinical governance on page 19). However, without a method of assessment it is difficult to demonstrate that quality standards are being met.

In the past, audit has often been used as the main tool for assessing quality. Although it is an important aspect of clinical governance, its inherent weakness is that it can only give an indication of the quality of what is being measured, and many important aspects of quality care cannot be measured by audit. Furthermore, audit undertaken in isolation from other tools of quality assessment can result in a mere academic exercise that has very little practical relevance.

Measurements of local performance against accepted 'gold standards' should provide a drive towards improving services. Although continual improvement of standards is a central tenet of the Government's definition of clinical governance, it is often difficult to achieve. Vital elements of the drive towards these improved standards are a multiprofessional team approach to both primary healthcare and organisational issues.

Multiprofessional approach

Modern primary healthcare is based on the primary healthcare team rather than on the individual GP. It is recognised that all members of the team, including receptionists, practice and community nurses, doctors, practice managers and other healthcare professionals attached to the team, play a vital role in the delivery of high-quality care. Good communication, mutual respect and teamworking skills are all key areas that need to be cultivated and maintained through a culture of openness and shared goals for the effective working of primary care teams. Governance activity undertaken by and considering only the work of a single professional group is unlikely to be effective. Quality control needs to involve all members of the team, and the standards and goals that are set need to be agreed by all team members. Failure of the whole team to agree on a governance strategy, and lack of clear ownership of the individual components as they affect different team members, will lead to poor outcomes and will breed a culture of suspicion and resentment. Larger practices will benefit from having a representative of each professional group in their governance team. In smaller practices this may not be possible, but wide consultation on governance issues among team members is still vital.

Organisational issues

As delivery of services by organisations – from health to public transport, and from Social Services to policing – has become increasingly complex, it has become clear how problems (and unfortunately sometimes disasters) are rarely the fault of a single individual, but usually involve a collective failure of the organisation and its management. There are frequent high-profile examples of these failures in national news stories. Complexity theory is useful for helping us to understand how these problems occur, since it illustrates how very large effects are normally produced by a series of small changes which may in themselves seem quite insignificant.

Primary care teams will need to examine their organisational and managerial procedures as part of clinical governance, and to consider how these impact upon the delivery of services to their patients. Management needs to encourage and enable multiprofessional teamworking by providing staff support, appraisal and investment in education and staff professional development. Primary care teams have the advantage of their relatively small size leading to potentially high levels of adaptability and close working relationships between staff, thereby fostering a healthy teamworking culture. Organisations and teams will function best if they are able to *learn about how they can most effectively learn*, a process termed the 'learning organisation'. What is effective for one practice team may not be effective for another. Small teams and organisations can benefit from the principles of 'action research' in facilitating evidence-based, purposeful and well-described development.

Tools of clinical governance

Although the definition of clinical governance is straightforward, the concept of what clinical governance involves in practice and how it is performed has caused much confusion. It is important to understand at the outset that clinical governance is not one single, clearly defined activity, but rather it consists of a 'pick-and-mix' selection of tools. How a practice goes about the task of clinical governance depends on where they are starting, the issue that they are aiming to address, and what resources they have available. It is important to stress that clinical governance is not an individual activity or a paper exercise, but rather it is a process that involves the whole team and includes a range of activities designed to lead to an improved service.

The range of clinical governance activities may include the following:

• implementing evidence-based practice
• auditing processes or outcomes
• risk management
• continuous professional development
• significant event auditing
• dealing with and learning from complaints
• patient and carer opinions
• teambuilding
• communication within and between organisations
• dealing with poor performance.

This list is not exhaustive, and several of these activities may be combined in a single clinical governance programme.

Palliative care and clinical governance

Palliative care provides an excellent opportunity for clinical governance. As an important aspect of cancer care, it falls within one of the areas of national importance defined by the Government. Furthermore, good palliative care is important for patients with congestive cardiac failure, and it is specifically highlighted within

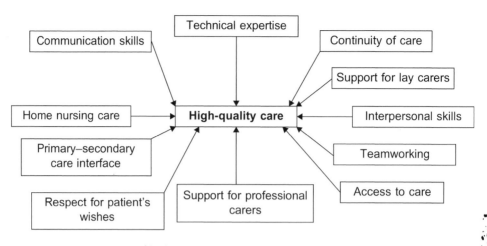

Figure 2.2 Components of high-quality palliative care.

the National Service Framework (NSF) for coronary heart disease, another national priority area.

Provision of good palliative care requires attention to many organisational, procedural, multidisciplinary and clinical areas (*see* Figure 2.2), all of which need a high degree of co-ordination. They cannot be assumed to function effectively within a practice or primary care team without clear evidence.

Implementing evidence-based practice

The evidence base for palliative care is not as clearly defined as in other areas of medicine. Traditional research methods such as the randomised controlled trial (RCT) are problematic, and ethical objections to research in palliative care have been raised. Recruitment is often slow, attrition rates are high and there is difficulty in controlling for confounding factors, since patients may have multiple problems and be receiving varying treatments. There is also difficulty in defining reliable outcome measures, especially for quality of life. Consequently, palliative medicine often relies on evidence taken from other disciplines (e.g. chronic pain management), with evidence of effectiveness in the palliative care setting relying on case series and non-experimental studies. The practice of palliative care has to be highly adaptable to individual and occasionally rare clinical problems, and it often requires a high level of innovation. In many of these complex situations, standard evidence from RCTs is of questionable relevance.

Many regions have developed guidelines for standard symptom control based on current practice. Specialists and generalists with special experience in palliative care are generally jointly responsible for the development of guidelines, making them relevant to the local situation. A valuable focus for clinical governance in palliative care could be 'getting guidelines into practice' (*see* Example 2.1).

Example 2.1

River Street Medical Practice has three partners. The newest partner, Dr Thomas, has taken the lead on clinical governance for the practice. He was a medical officer in a local hospice when he was on his GP registrar rotation. He notices when he visits one of Dr Jefferson's patients on a Saturday morning that he is on a rather bizarre combination of analgesics for pain from bone secondaries from a renal carcinoma. He decides that rather than speak directly to Dr Jefferson at this stage, he will survey all of the patients in the practice with a diagnosis of metastatic carcinoma on the practice computer. He finds that it seems that not only Dr Jefferson, but also his other partner Dr Forbes, uses analgesics in a rather erratic way.

At their next practice meeting, when they are discussing clinical govern-ance issues he brings up the subject of guidelines for symptom control in palliative care patients. Both of his partners reveal that they were not aware that local guidelines existed, but expressed interest in looking at them, as they both found palliative care a difficult area. Dr Thomas arranges for Dr Dale, a Macmillan palliative care GP facilitator, and the Macmillan nurse attached to the practice to visit for an educational meeting, which will qualify for PGEA points. The neighbouring Lakeside Medical Group also join them, invited by Dr Thomas, who is in a young principals' group with Dr Patel, a partner at Lakeside.

Dr Dale explains that the guidelines were put together by a group including himself and the local hospice medical director. Both practices are impressed. They decide to adopt the guidelines and arrange that each doctor will have a copy in his consulting room and in his 'doctor's bag'. Dr Dale is asked by Dr Gregson from the Lakeside Medical Group, who is also the local clinical tutor, whether they can discuss the possibility of arranging an after-noon session on symptom control at the local postgraduate centre.

Risk management

The identification of areas of risk for special attention and study is of great importance. Areas that are appropriate for risk management include communica-tion, practice procedures, interdisciplinary working, prescribing and therapeutics, and patient referrals.

Terminally ill patients need continuity of care. Research has shown that patients may see up to 30 different doctors during a period of one year when suffering from advanced cancer. Not only does this cause problems with the flow of information to the various professionals involved in patient care, but also it can be bewildering for the patient and their carers, and can cause confusion in their minds if different professionals give them different explanations. Receiving personal continuity of care from their GP may ameliorate this problem, and they will be greatly reassured by the personal interest and attention that are shown towards them.

Unfortunately, with the multitude of calls that come through surgery reception, patients or their carers may find it difficult to see their usual doctor. This is an area where a risk management strategy may improve access of patients to their usual doctor. A system may be introduced to ensure that receptionists know which patients are terminally ill, and doctors within the practice accept that they will give priority to dealing with these patients should they call (*see* Examples 2.2 and 2.3).

Example 2.2 (part of this example is adapted from an article in *GP* published on 8 October 1999)

Susie Rees, the district nurse attached to Brook Street Surgery, a nine-doctor practice, has received several comments from patients indicating that they had difficulty in arranging visits from the GPs at the surgery. Her district nursing colleagues who also work with Brook Street Surgery confirm that patients have made similar comments to them. She approaches Dr Jones, the clinical governance lead at the practice, to express her concern that there might be a problem. Dr Jones brings up the problem at a practice meeting where the practice team members discuss the situation. They decide to investigate the process whereby calls for visits are received by receptionists at the practice.

Liz James, the senior receptionist, explains how they have difficulty in identifying patients with special needs, and how they also have difficulties with taking calls in the morning, especially with the increasing numbers of patients who are phoning up for repeat prescriptions. Dr Evans, the GP registrar, remembers that she saw a report in a GP magazine about a practice which had introduced a colour-coding system to identify terminally ill patients. Patients' names were placed on a board in reception so that the reception staff could clearly see which patients needed to be given high priority for seeing a doctor. It also helped to remind staff which patients needed regular visiting even if they had not formally requested a visit. Sid Granger, the practice manager, agreed to investigate this. On finding that the practice described in the article was an NHS Beacon site and was only an hour away, they decided to arrange a visit to investigate their system.

As a result of the visit, they introduced a similar system tailored to their own practice, and they decided to ask patients and their carers whether they had experienced any difficulty in requesting a visit. They also decided to use a separate telephone line for repeat prescription requests, received by a dedicated receptionist who would be doing clerical work while awaiting these calls. In addition, they asked the district nurses to give them any further feedback which they received from patients.

Example 2.3

A complaint was received at Goodnight Doc, the local out-of-hours co-operative. It was from the daughter of an elderly patient with end-stage prostate cancer called Jim Furness. His wife called the co-operative for a visit and was asked if the patient could come down to the on-call centre. When she said that he was too unwell to do this, they were told that they would have to wait for at least 3 hours before a doctor could see them. Jim was in such pain that his daughter called for an ambulance. He was taken to the local Accident and Emergency department, but died soon after arrival. Dr George, the patient's GP, had already spoken to the medical manager about this situation and they agreed that it should be investigated.

They reviewed their procedures for dealing with telephone calls and found that the receptionists did not have clear instructions for dealing with this type of situation. It also seemed that it was rare for any information to be sent in from practices with regard to terminally ill patients. However, when they talked to individual doctors, they all said that they routinely sent information to the co-operative with regard to their terminally ill patients.

The co-operative clinical governance committee decided to conduct an audit over a period of one month to see how often information about terminally ill patients was received. They asked the night district nursing service to identify all of the patients registered with co-operative members who had an estimated prognosis of three months or less. The audit revealed that for those patients who were identified, only 20% of the practices with whom these patients were registered had sent any communication to the co-operative.

The committee, with the help of Dr Dale, the GP palliative care facilitator, designed a fax form prompting specific information which the co-operative should receive. The membership, on being presented with the audit results, unanimously agreed to use the fax form. The receptionists were also given specific training in how to deal with these calls. Six months later the audit was repeated, and it was found that fax forms had been received for 60% of terminally ill patients.

Computers in risk management

Terminally ill patients often receive a plethora of drugs to control their symptoms. It is widely accepted that patients who are started on opioid analgesics may need to take laxatives to prevent the onset of constipation. However, this is often forgotten, especially in general practice where many drug interactions and side-effects need to be remembered. Most practices use computer systems to generate prescriptions, so it is possible for drug warnings to be flashed on to the computer screen should certain drugs be prescribed. A message reading 'Prescribe laxative?' or some similar prompt could help to reduce the risk of an opioid being prescribed without a laxative.

Audit

Audit is a very important tool for clinical governance. It can be especially powerful when used together with other tools such as risk management or significant event auditing, or as a baseline assessment. This reduces the risk of audit being performed merely to fulfil an obligation to be involved in running audits – a criticism that is often made of the 'audit culture'. Linking audits in with other governance tools to answer a specific question is likely to produce important results, rather than being merely a theoretical exercise.

Audit should be performed to test performance against previously set standards. The results should then be used to encourage change. All professionals involved in delivering this particular service should agree upon the changes. Once changes have been made, the standards should be re-examined. Were they originally set too low (was quality higher than expected)? Or were they set too high (do we need to take a more realistic look at what is achievable)? The process of reassessing standards is then followed by a repeat of the audit cycle (*see* Figure 2.3) to measure the effect of the changes made (*see* Example 2.4, and also Example 2.3).

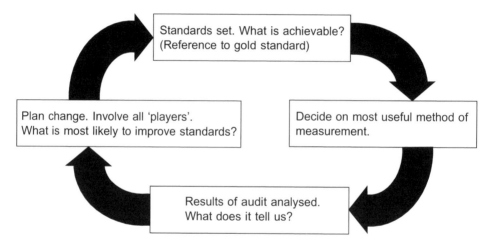

Figure 2.3 The audit cycle.

Example 2.4

A newly set up multiprofessional group monitoring the Hospice at Home service (*see* Example 2.5) became concerned that there seemed to be a lack of continuity when patients were discharged from the inpatient hospice. They spoke to a number of GPs about the situation. Several GPs felt that the discharge summaries which they received from the hospice were poor, and they were often not informed about patients being discharged at an early stage.

The multiprofessional group approached the hospice medical director, who agreed to meet with the group to discuss the situation. At the meeting it was decided that together they would design a discharge summary form which the hospice could use, and that for a period of six months all discharge summaries would be accompanied by an audit form for GPs to report back on the quality of information received. The hospice nursing director also agreed that the senior nurse on duty on the morning of discharge would telephone the patient's practice to inform them of the discharge.

Significant event analysis

In practice, the unexpected often happens. Sometimes mistakes may occur or the outcome may be significantly different to what was expected. Significant or critical event analysis is a process whereby unexpected events are examined to discover what can be learned from them. The process is used extensively in the airline industry to examine 'near misses'. A near disaster will often precede a disaster. If we can learn the lesson of the 'significant event', we may be able to put into effect changes to prevent a recurrence that has a potentially more serious outcome. We may also discover other issues that need to be investigated further (e.g. organisational failure, poor inter-professional communication or lack of clarity in guidelines).

Areas of palliative care that are likely to be fruitful for significant event auditing include the following:

* difficulties in communication
* problems arising between primary care and specialist palliative care teams
* inappropriate use of drugs
* failure to diagnose emergencies (e.g. hypercalcaemia or spinal cord compression).

There is a natural tendency to try to forget mistakes or even to cover them up, particularly within a 'blame culture' where someone is sought out to take full responsibility for an adverse outcome. Significant event auditing does not work well in such a culture. At present, within the UK there is a call for increased openness in public organisations, which is occurring in tandem with a wish to 'name and shame' those organisations and individuals who seem to have failed. These two cultures appear to be directly opposed, and it remains to be seen whether we can develop a 'no-blame' culture in healthcare organisations which will foster the use of this potentially powerful tool (*see* Example 2.1).

Complaints

According to one UK Secretary of State for Health, complaints should be treasured as jewels. A London GP was rather more sanguine when he suggested in a general practice periodical that GPs should treat complaints in the same way that inner-city GPs treated parking tickets! Whatever our feelings about complaints – and no one likes to receive them – they can be used as a starting point for significant event analysis.

All practices are required to have a system for dealing with complaints so that local resolution of the problem can occur if possible. If there is some substance to the complaint, it is usual to state as part of the apology to the complainant that steps are being taken to ensure that similar failings do not recur. Clearly, this should lead directly to clinical governance activity.

Complaints do occur in the area of palliative care (*see* Example 2.3), although they are not common. They most commonly arise as a result of poor communication, failure to visit, or failure to make a diagnosis until the terminal stage of a disease has been reached. Although few formal complaints are made, it is not uncommon for patients and their carers to express concern or anger to other professionals. These 'unexpressed complaints' may be just as effectively used in clinical governance (*see* Example 2.2).

Continuing professional development (CPD)

All healthcare professions need to be involved in CPD in order to update and improve their knowledge and skills. One criticism of the current Postgraduate Education Allowance (PGEA) is that doctors tend to undergo educational activities in areas in which they are already proficient, while ignoring areas of greater personal need. One increasingly popular solution to this problem is for doctors to keep learning portfolios, so that they can demonstrate the educational activities in which they have been involved and formulate plans for further professional development. These portfolios can undergo peer review by a GP tutor or mentor to ensure that CPD is broadly based and tailored to the clinician's needs. These portfolios may well form one of the features of professional revalidation to be introduced in the UK within the next two years.

Identification of the need for CPD activity in a particular area may result from other clinical governance activity (e.g. as a consequence of audit or critical event analysis) (*see* Example 2.1).

Communication within and between teams

Good palliative care needs to be truly multidisciplinary. Much of the daily follow-up and care undertaken with the terminally ill involves district nurses, who see palliative care as an important aspect of their work, as do patients and their carers. The GP needs to be closely involved with the care of his or her patients in order to facilitate management decisions and provide ongoing continuity of medical care. The situation can change rapidly during the terminal stage of a patient's illness, and without regular contact the GP can soon be out of touch with his or her patient's condition and care. Clear procedures for communication within practice teams, such as regular clinical meetings between GPs and district nurses, can facilitate communication. There also needs to be mutual respect among different professionals, with an acknowledgement of one another's skills and the limits to one's own skills. Teams in which there is mutual suspicion and lack of communication are likely to function poorly, to the detriment of patient care.

The primary care team is central to the care of the terminally ill, but specialist teams often have a close relationship with the patient and carer. Community clinical nurse specialists (Macmillan nurses) and 'Hospice at Home' nurses may visit the patient at home. The patient may attend a hospice day-care unit and be admitted to the hospice inpatient unit for symptom control or respite care. With many different professionals and teams being involved, there is great potential for communication problems leading to problems with continuity of care, and confusion for the patient and relatives. Good verbal and written communication is essential in order to maintain continuity of care. Clinical governance activity between primary and secondary care teams is likely to identify areas of weakness in communication, which can then be addressed (*see* Example 2.4).

Involvement of patients and carers

Ultimately, the most important test of quality for a service is whether or not it meets the needs of patients and their carers. One major problem in palliative care is that needs do vary, and what one patient or carer regards as a good feature of a service, another might consider to be less satisfactory.

It is possible to involve patients and carers by using a questionnaire, forming a patient/carer group or conducting an interview study, focusing on a particular service or aspect of care. Terminally ill patients and their carers are a difficult group to survey, as it is a stressful time for the whole family, and meaningful questionnaires are difficult to design for this group, although validated questionnaires such as the Palliative Outcome Scale (POS) may be useful in some circumstances. It is also especially difficult to form a representative group of terminally ill patients. Interview studies are labour- and cost-intensive, and are often conducted with carers several months after the patient's death. However, they may provide a more complete picture than questionnaires of the problems faced by terminally ill patients (*see* Example 2.5).

Example 2.5

The South Forest PCT faces a dilemma. With the creation of the PCT last year, they inherited all of the community services from the old South Forest Community NHS Trust. Along with this came the 10-bed hospice and Hospice-at-Home service. GP members of the Professional Executive Committee (PEC) seem divided about the benefit of the Hospice-at-Home service, with about half of the members regarding it as a useful service, and the other half feeling that it is neither useful nor cost-effective. They have discussed the situation with the clinical governance committee of the PCT, and it was decided that they would speak to the 'primary care research unit' at Forest University, which they know has an interest in community palliative care.

The research unit explains to the PCT that there was no research which showed that Hospice-at-Home services definitely allowed more patients to die at home, but there were methodological problems involved in attempting to subject this type of service to a clinical trial. Working with the PCT, the research unit arranges with one of their academic registrars to perform a research project where the registrar would conduct interviews with bereaved carers (both those who had received Hospice-at-Home care and those who had not). High levels of satisfaction were found in the Hospice-at-Home group, while the relatives of patients who had not received this care also expressed high levels of satisfaction, but seemed more likely to make negative comments, especially about some aspects of care being lacking. In response to a parallel questionnaire that was sent to all district nurses, there was a high level of agreement that the Hospice-at-Home service was useful. Some district nurses expressed concern that some of the GPs with whom they worked did not use the service, and it was felt that some admissions would have been avoidable if the Hospice-at-Home service had been used.

As the service was clearly popular with carers and district nurses, it was decided to continue with it, but to set up a multiprofessional group to monitor the service.

Conclusion

Clinical governance is a process rather than an event. All of the tools for clinical governance should be used in an integrated manner with clear goals to ensure that the process leads to the identification of problems and a drive towards high-quality care. All NHS trusts and authorities have a statutory duty to perform clinical governance and to identify a lead professional. In primary care, most clinical governance activity will need to be devolved to individual practices and teams, with all members of the primary care team being involved in the process. Within these teams, a named professional or a group given specific responsibility for its organisation should lead clinical governance.

Palliative care is an important aspect of primary care, and it can only be performed well by a multidisciplinary team and when there is good communication both within the primary care team and across the primary care–specialist interface. It is also an important aspect of several National Service Frameworks (NSFs) which form a focus for current clinical governance activity. The full range of clinical governance tools is useful for ensuring high-quality palliative care.

Reference

1 Department of Health (1998) *A First-Class Service.* Department of Health, London.

Further reading

• Department of Health (1999) *Clinical Governance in the New NHS.* Department of Health, London.

- Roland M, Holden J and Campbell S (1998) *Quality Assessment for General Practice: supporting clinical governance in primary care groups.* National Primary Care Research and Development Centre, Manchester (available at www.npcrdc.man.ac.uk).

Clinical governance in primary care: *British Medical Journal* articles

- Allen P (2000) Accountability for clinical governance: developing collective responsibility for quality in primary care. *BMJ.* **321**: 608–11.
- Huntington J, Gillam S and Rosen R (2000) Organisational development for clinical governance. *BMJ.* **321**: 679–82.
- McColl A and Roland M (2000) Knowledge and information for clinical governance. *BMJ.* **321**: 871–4.
- Pringle M (2000) Participating in clinical governance. *BMJ.* **321**: 737–40.
- Rosen R (2000) Improving quality in the changing world of primary care. *BMJ.* **321**: 551–4.

Other articles

- Davies H and Nutley SM (2000) Developing learning organisations in the new NHS. *BMJ.* **320**: 998–1001.
- Hearn J and Higginson I (1999) Development and validation of a core outcome measure for palliative care: the Palliative Care Outcome Scale. *Qual Health Care.* **8**: 219–27.

Useful websites

NHS Clinical Governance Support Team; www.cgsupport.org
National Primary Care Research and Development Centre; www.npcrdc.man.ac.uk
Clinical Governance Bulletin (free online journal); www.rsm.ac.uk/pub/cgb.htm
Wisdom (electronic approach to postgraduate education); www.wisdom.org.uk
National Electronic Library for Health; www.nelh.nhs.uk
National Institute for Clinical Excellence (NICE); www.nice.org.uk
National Council for Hospice and Specialist Palliative Care; www.hospice-spc-council.org.uk
NHS Beacon website; www.nhsbeacon.org.uk

CHAPTER 3

Communication with the dying and their loved ones

Joanne Fisher and Mandy Barnett

Introduction

The diagnosis of any illness, in particular a life-threatening illness, is one of the most emotionally distressing events that a person may experience in their lifetime. The distress caused by such a diagnosis can be reduced by open communication between patients, health professionals and the patient's family and friends. Open communication enables patients to discuss their concerns, and this has been shown to reduce anxiety, promote adjustment and decrease the isolation that patients often feel when suffering from a life-threatening illness. However, it is just this type of illness that can lead to difficulties in communication. For example, doctors often feel inadequately prepared to discuss the issues associated with life-threatening illness, and the patient's relatives and friends may avoid discussing the subject. This chapter explores communication processes between primary health-care professionals, patients and their loved ones, and suggests communication techniques that may be employed to improve dialogue for the benefit of all.

Anxiety about the possibility that one may have a life-threatening illness

The diagnostic path of illness commonly elicits anxiety. Events such as medical investigations, waiting for the results, diagnosis and fear of recurrence are particularly anxiety provoking. Anxiety is a common reaction to uncertainty, and may produce both psychological and physical symptoms. Common psychological symptoms include worry, irritability, restlessness and insomnia. Physical symptoms include palpitations, sweating and nausea. In order to minimise anxiety, it is important to ensure that patients undergo any investigations as soon as possible and that the results are made available and discussed quickly.

Confirmation of the diagnosis
Telling the patient

When the diagnosis has been confirmed, it is important to inform the patient. Recently there has been a move towards greater openness in the communication of information about life-threatening illness between doctors and patients. This has been demonstrated by an increase in the number of doctors who prefer to inform their patients of their diagnosis. For example, Novac[1] replicated a study conducted in 1962 which explored doctors' attitude to informing patients about their cancer diagnosis, and found a reversal in approach, with 98% of doctors informing patients of their cancer diagnosis. Similar recent surveys in the UK reported that 95% of GPs always or often tell patients about a cancer diagnosis,[2] and that patients desire information about their illness. A study of the information needs of patients diagnosed with cancer in the UK reported that most people with cancer want to be given all of the available information about their illness.[3] However, some patients, especially those with a poor prognosis, may not want to know all the details. Therefore it is perhaps appropriate to keep asking 'Is there anything else you would like to know?'. Research has shown that healthcare professionals find it easier to treat and care for patients if they know their diagnosis,[4] and open communication is associated with the following benefits for patients:[5]

- clearer information
- participation in decision making
- psychological support
- decreased anxiety
- preparation for death
- acceptance.

Patients also need relevant information about their illness if they are to make informed decisions about their treatment and care. For example, Meredith[3] found that patients wished to know:

- the name of their illness
- whether the illness was cancer
- the treatment options and side-effects
- the likelihood of cure.

This is consistent with the view expressed in the General Medical Council's guidelines (*see* Box 3.1).[6]

Box 3.1   General Medical Council guidelines: the right to know

Right to know
Diagnosis
Prognosis
Time scale
Treatment options
Costs where relevant
Outcomes of treatment
Side-effects of treatment

At present many doctors consider that their training has inadequately prepared them for communicating bad news to patients. One study found that almost one-third of GP registrars had not received formal training in 'breaking bad news,' and that 94% avoided breaking bad news during a consultation.[7] In addition, GP registrars cited the following reasons for failure to break bad news during a consultation. They were afraid of:

• upsetting the patient
• causing more harm than good
• having to answer difficult questions
• having to handle difficult emotional states.

Not being informed about their illness is the commonest complaint that patients make about the medical profession.[8] Open communication is therefore important for both doctors and patients[9] (*see* Box 3.2).

Box 3.2   Functions of communication

Maintain trust
Reduce uncertainty
Prevent unrealistic expectations
Allow patients to adjust
Prevent a conspiracy of silence

Although it can be argued that breaking bad news insensitively or inadequately can lead to poor long-term adjustment for patients and their relatives,[10] the research to support this notion is limited. Nevertheless, doctors who are anxious when breaking bad news are perceived less positively in terms of their effectiveness. Buckman[11] argues that the difficulties experienced by doctors when breaking bad news are due to a complex interaction of social, patient, professional and personal factors (*see* Box 3.3).[3]

Box 3.3 Difficulties encountered during communication with dying patients

Social factors
 Denial of death
 Lack of experience
 High expectations of health
 Materialism
 The changing role of religion

Patient factors
 Fears of dying
 Anxiety about treatment
 Psychological effects
 Family and friends
 Finances, social status, job

Professional factors
 Fears of eliciting a reaction
 Fears of being blamed
 Sympathetic pain
 Minimal education
 Concerns about saying 'I don't know'
 Anxiety about expressing emotions
 Concerns about one's own mortality

How to tell the patient

Although it is more commonly the task of secondary care specialists, GPs are inevitably involved in breaking bad news. There are no universally agreed guidelines on how bad news should be broken, but there is a general consensus,[12] and a number of protocols have been proposed.[9,13,14] The use of such guidelines can improve the 'breaking bad news' consultation for both doctor and patient.[11]

Table 3.1 Guidelines for breaking bad news[9]

Preparation

- Know all the facts.
- Invite the patient to bring someone with them (a relative or friend).
- Set time aside, avoid interruptions, introduce yourself, sit down, and have tissues available.

What is known

The patient may deny having much insight into their illness, so try to elicit what they know before explaining. Asking the patient for a narrative of recent events may lead to disclosure of current knowledge, such as:

- level of understanding
- main concerns
- beliefs
- expectations for the future.

Is more information wanted?

- If the patient asks for more information, offer a warning shot.
- If the patient is unsure whether they want more information, discuss the pros and cons.
- If the patient declines more information, respect their wish and do not impose more information, but facilitate questioning at a later date.

Allow denial

- Denial is a coping mechanism that is unlikely to be permanently adopted.
- Never give unrequested information, as it can cause anxiety or anger.

Give a warning shot

- A warning shot allows consideration of feelings.
- A warning shot gives the patient time to consider whether they want more information.
- Use the patient's own words to explore what they understand.

Explain

- This will reduce the information gap.
- The aim is to reduce uncertainty without causing fear.
- Provide a narrative of events.
- Avoid the use of medical jargon.
- Check the patient's understanding.
- Be optimistic.
- Deal with the patient's concerns.

Elicit concerns

- This allows verbalisation and enables the patient to clarify and prioritise their concerns.
- Avoid giving premature reassurance.
- Avoid excessive explanations.

Encourage ventilation of feelings

This is a therapeutic part of the dialogue.

- Acknowledge feelings.
- Verbalise feelings.
- Hear one's own words.
- Name the emotion.
- This fosters a sense of control.

Summary

- Summarise concerns.
- Plan treatment.
- Foster hope.
- Ask if there is anything else that the patient would like to discuss.

Offer availability

Availability is important.

- Some of the details may not be remembered.
- Patients may think of subsequent questions and bring a list.
- Emotional adjustment takes time.
- It is helpful to talk to family members and friends.
- Over time, further information may be required.

In addition, it is important to document the consultation fully in the patient's notes.

Document the consultation[15]

The consultation should be fully documented in the patient's records, and the following information should be included:

- patient's name
- date and place of consultation
- who was present
- what the patient has been told
- the patient's response
- treatment options, if these were discussed
- management strategy
- list of healthcare professionals to be informed/contacted.

Baile and Buckman[16] have developed a useful mnemonic (SPIKES) for communicating medical information (*see* Box 3.4).

Box 3.4   The SPIKES protocol for breaking bad news[16]

S   **Setting** and listening skills
P   Patient's **perception**
I   **Invitation** from patient to give information
K   **Knowledge** – giving medical facts
E   **Explore** emotions and empathise as patient responds
S   **Strategy** and **summary**

A recording of the consultation in the form of written notes and/or audiotapes has been used by some clinicians in an attempt to improve communication. Some research studies have shown that patients find this approach useful, both as a means of assimilating information and as a method of disseminating information to relatives and friends.[17] However, one study has found that patients with a poor prognosis found the audiotapes increased distress.[18]

Breaking bad news is a difficult area of clinical practice, causing doctors anxiety which in some cases leads to the avoidance of breaking such news. The application of the measures outlined above should help to improve the consultation for both the giver and the receiver of bad news. Participation in a course designed to improve skills in breaking bad news is recommended, and has been found to be beneficial.[7]

Supportive care and communication for those who are dying

The final phase of the illness may be stressful and difficult for the patient and their family and friends. The fear that surrounds death often leads the patient's family and friends to avoid confronting the issue because:

- they are afraid of upsetting the patient
- they are afraid of their emotional response to the imminent death
- for some death is a taboo subject.

Such barriers make open discussion of issues and emotions concerning the patient and their family and friends difficult. There may also be mismatch of communication preference between patients and their family and friends. Some may prefer to discuss these issues openly, while others will prefer not to confront such issues. This mismatch may not be very supportive and may require intervention. In addition, opportunities to talk openly may be further reduced in the final phase of a terminal illness, as the patient's social network shrinks because:

- the patient is afraid of upsetting or depressing their family or friends
- the patient may be concerned about how their family and friends will cope in the final phase
- the patient may wish to have space to come to terms with their feelings.

Fear of death and the process of dying is common, because of the lack of control and the uncertainty that exists about the patient's death, which may be painful and/or undignified. It is important to elicit the patient's concerns regarding such issues. Pain can be worsened by distress, fear, anger, depression, uncertainty and guilt. Discussion of a feared terminal event, such as a haemorrhage (haemoptysis or haematemesis) or respiratory distress, with the patient and/or their relatives may prove useful. For example, it may help to discuss with the patient the likelihood of the feared event occurring, and in cases where such an event is possible, discussion of its management can often lead to a more realistic view of it.

Patients' adjustment to dying

The knowledge that death is imminent has a profound effect on the patient, their family and friends and healthcare professionals, and subsequently people will behave differently towards the patient. People adjust to the knowledge that they are dying in different ways and at different speeds. Kübler-Ross,[19] a psychiatrist, investigated people's reactions to dying and proposed that they progressed through five psychological stages in adjusting to death (*see* Box 3.5).

Box 3.5 Stages of adjustment to dying[19]

Denial and isolation
Anger
Bargaining
Depression
Acceptance

Denial
This is a common initial reaction to the knowledge that the illness is terminal. The duration of this stage will vary, although some people may get 'stuck' in this phase.

Anger
Anger can be a distressing reaction for family and friends, who may become the target of the patient's anger, as too may healthcare professionals.

Bargaining
Bargaining is an attempt to postpone the inevitable. This reaction may take the form of a pact.

Depression
Depression may result from the knowledge that the illness cannot be stayed, as evidenced by worsening symptoms.

Acceptance
Finally, the stage of acceptance is reached. However, some patients do not accept the prospect of death. During this stage the patient may disengage, maintaining just a small network of family and friends.

Although the stage model has provided insights into the process of adjustment to death, there is little evidence for the existence of progressive stages of adjustment. Kübler-Ross interviewed patients at different stages of their illness. Thus the stages that she describes may be emotional responses that are experienced by dying patients, rather than the 'normal' progression towards acceptance. Kübler-Ross also failed to take into account the influence of variables such as gender, age, ethnicity, culture and relational provision in her account. Even so, the model is widely known, and family and friends may be distressed if the patient does not progress through the expected stages. In contrast, Buckman[11] categorises patient behaviour to provide an indication of adjustment (*see* Table 3.2).

Table 3.2   Responses to dying[11]

Adaptive	*Maladaptive*
Humour	Guilt
Denial	Pathological denial
Abstract anger	Anger directed against helpers
Anger directed against disease	Collapse
Crying	Anxiety
Fear	The impossible 'quest'
Fulfilling an ambition	Unrealistic hope
Realistic hope	Despair
Sexual drive	Manipulation
Bargaining	Suicidal

Although no one model is yet able to account for all of the behaviours observed in this process, a general framework may be useful for explaining people's behaviour at this time.

Talking to the patient's relatives

The experience of a life-threatening illness affects the whole family. Communication with the patient's relatives is important, as they often form part of the care team, and because of their privileged knowledge they may be able to advise on issues concerning the patient. Therefore communication with the relatives is a dynamic process in which they act as providers and receivers of information.

Some relatives prefer that their loved ones are not told the truth, or that they are presented with a modified version of the facts. Relatives often claim that the truth would have a deleterious effect, causing the patient to suffer from depression or to give up the will to fight. Under the Access to Health Records Act (1990), doctors are permitted some freedom to withhold information if they believe that it may be harmful to patients (i.e. 'information likely to cause serious harm to the physical or mental health of the patient or of any other individual'). Relatives often take this approach in the belief that they are protecting their loved ones. However, the presence of such barriers may have an adverse effect on the patient. Kastenbaum[20] found that many patients know they are dying, and the lack of open communication only serves to increase their sense of isolation as they approach death unsupported.

In addition, relatives may ask for information about the patient, such as the diagnosis, prognosis and treatment care, without the patient's knowledge. Although doctors have a duty to maintain confidentiality with regard to patient information, this is not absolute. Doctors may disclose information about their patient to others under certain circumstances (e.g. if the patient gives their consent to the disclosure or if the doctor can justify the disclosure). The General Medical Council provides guidelines on the unconsented disclosure of information that:

• is justified in the public interest
• is essential to protect the patient or someone else from risk of death or serious harm
• relates to patients who are not competent.

Obtaining consent to disclose information to relatives is good practice. The doctor must first discuss with the patient how much information will be disclosed and to whom. If the patient withholds their consent, then the doctor must be able to justify any disclosure. Research has shown that the majority of people are opposed to doctors disclosing information without their consent.[21] However, in certain circumstances, disclosure without consent might be appropriate (e.g. if the patient was incapacitated or unconscious, or if the relationship between the doctor and the family was close). Most of the study participants thought that it was beneficial for doctors to disclose consented information to families, as this promoted openness.

Finally, it is important to consider that relatives may also need support and are often reluctant to ask for help in coping because they feel that the patient comes first.

Talking to children about their illness

Any discussion with a child about his or her illness, especially when active treatment is not possible, is a difficult and distressing task. Some parents are unable to talk openly with their sick child, yet children often have an understanding of their illness and its possible outcome. The Association for Children with Life-Threatening or Terminal Conditions and their Families (ACT) suggests that discussions with children should be 'sensitive and appropriate to age and understanding', as it is known that children vary in their level of understanding about death (e.g. some children under five believe that death is temporary).[22] Discussion with children about their illness enables them to have an input into decisions about their care. Communication is not restricted to verbal discussion, and may include drawings, play and stories to try to communicate what is happening.

Talking to children about their parent's illness

In general, the task of breaking bad news about a parent's illness to a child or children is left to parents. However, many parents do not disclose a life-threatening illness to their children even if they are undergoing surgery or chemotherapy.[23] Parents often believe that by not disclosing their diagnosis they are protecting their children from anxiety and distress.[21,23] Yet research indicates that children's anxiety levels are lower when there is open communication within families.[24]

Many patients would welcome advice on disclosing information about their illness to their children. In addition, studies have shown that parents wanted children to have the opportunity to talk to health professionals directly.[23] It is recommended that parents are offered help in disclosing information about their illness to their children. Such help should take account of the child's age and understanding, and family communication system, as well as the parent's own feeling about their illness and the parent's ability to cope with the child's feelings about their illness.

Box 3.6   Summary of communication with a patient's family

An important part of the patient care
Receivers and providers of information
'Victims' other than the patient
Parents sometimes need advice about talking to children
Individual circumstances should always be considered

Advance directives

Advance directives (ADs) (also known as 'living wills') are documents that enable patients to specify their consent or dissent to medical treatment prospectively, in case they later become incapable of making such decisions.[25] In law, if a patient becomes incapable of making decisions, it is assumed that they would consent to life-preserving measures. ADs take a number of different forms, including requesting or authorising treatment, refusing treatment, stating general values and preferences, naming an advocate, or a combination of any of these.[25]

Advance directives have been advocated as a way of improving open communication between patients and health professionals and family and friends with regard to healthcare issues.[26] ADs relate to the decisions that individuals make about perceived future outcomes.[26] Research has suggested that the stability of such decisions changes as a function of illness severity and time. For example, Danis[27] found that although most future treatment preferences remained stable over a two-year period, people who had been hospitalised or involved in accidents or who had become immobile during this period were more likely to change their treatment preferences and favour more intervention treatment.

There is uncertainty about the legal standing of ADs.[28] The British Medical Association has issued guidelines on the current law and medical practice:

> It is a general point of law and medical practice that all adults have the right to consent to or refuse medical treatment. Advance statements are a means for patients to exercise that right by anticipating a time when they may lose the capacity to make or communicate a decision.[25]

However, not all ADs are legally binding. In those that are, 'the individual must have envisaged the type of situation which has subsequently arisen'.[25,29]

Although the format of ADs is not legally specified, the BMA has issued guidelines on the minimum elements that should be included (*see* Box 3.7).[25]

> **Box 3.7**   Checklist for writing an advance directive
>
> Full name
> Address
> Signature
> Witness signature
> Date drafted and reviewed
> A clear statement of wishes (either general or specific)
> Name and address of general practitioner
> Was advice sought from healthcare professionals?
> Name, address and telephone number of a nominated person, if any

Talking to the bereaved

Bereavement is the process of adaptation to loss. It can be challenging and may have adverse health consequences, including increased morbidity and mortality,[29] although the exact mechanism involved is unclear. Adverse health consequences may result from the commencement or exacerbation of behaviours that may lead to ill health, such as excess alcohol consumption.[30]

The bereavement process has been variously described,[31,32] and is commonly envisaged as stages through which the bereaved person progresses (*see* Box 3.8). These stages are not fixed, and many people oscillate between different stages, remain in one stage or experience several of the emotional stages simultaneously.

> **Box 3.8**   Stages in the bereavement process
>
> Shock, numbness, disbelief
> Acute distress, anger
> Disorganisation and despair
> Reorganisation, acceptance and resolution

Phase models of bereavement have a number of limitations. For example, the model assumes that distress is normal, so not becoming distressed might be an indication of pathological bereavement.

The bereaved may experience physical symptoms, including the following:

- breathing problems, tightness, shortness of breath
- anxiety
- lethargy
- feeling tense
- mental pain
- symptoms of the deceased person's illness.

The bereaved person may also experience some of the following:

1 seeing and hearing the deceased person
2 mistaking others for the deceased person
3 assuming characteristics of the deceased person, such as:

   • mannerisms
   • personality traits.

These symptoms may be raised as concerns. Over a period of time, which can be up to 12 months or longer, the bereaved person usually adjusts to their loss and returns to a normal pattern of behaviour. However, the effect of the loss may continue, although diminished, for some time – perhaps even years.

The pattern of behaviours described above is typical of uncomplicated grief. However, for some individuals the symptoms of bereavement may not lessen, and this may lead to complicated grief (also called 'pathological bereavement'). There is no universal definition of complicated grief. Some theorists focus on the time scale, whereas others focus on symptoms as indicators (e.g. intense and prolonged emotional experiences, social withdrawal or clinical depression). A number of risk factors for pathological bereavement have been identified[33] (*see* Box 3.9). Failure to resolve grief may require professional intervention. In order to help patients in the grief process and to detect complicated grief, doctors must employ basic communication skills to listen and demonstrate empathy.

Box 3.9   Risk factors for pathological bereavement

Poor support network
Sudden death
Poor coping strategies
Poor physical health
Young age

Support for the bereaved

Although not all bereaved people need or wish to have support at this time, a number of interventions have been suggested as being beneficial to the bereaved,[29] such as:

• self-help groups
• voluntary organisations
• counselling
• contact from the GP or another member of the primary healthcare team (visiting, sending a letter or card, or telephoning).[34]

Research has suggested that the degree of contact is related to the level of involvement with a dying patient, and GPs who were intensely involved with the dying patient were more likely to visit the bereaved, whereas GPs who were less deeply involved or not involved at all were less likely to make contact.[35] An ideal approach would enable all GP practices to utilise a bereavement worker whose role would be to make contact with bereaved patients and enable them to express their feelings.

Box 3.10   Summary

Bereavement is a challenging process.
Bereavement can have an adverse effect on health.
Phase models offer a guide for understanding the grief process.
Good communication skills are important.
A bereavement worker can facilitate the grieving process.

Conclusion

Communication with the dying represents a major aspect of palliative care, and the guidelines outlined in this chapter are not rigid, but change according to individual patients and their circumstances. Good and open communication can have benefits both for patients and their family and for health professionals.

References

1 Novack PH, Plumer R, Smith RL, Ochitill H, Morrow GR and Bennett JM (1979) Changes in physicians' attitudes towards telling the cancer patient. *JAMA*. **242**: 897–900.

2 Vassilas CA and Donaldson J (1988) Telling the truth: what do general practitioners say to patients with dementia or terminal cancer? *Br J Gen Pract*. **48**: 1081–2.

3 Meredith C, Symonds P, Webster L *et al.* (1996) Information needs of cancer patients in west Scotland: cross-sectional survey of patients' views. *BMJ*. **313**: 724–6.

4 Seale C (1991) Communication and awareness about death: a study of a random sample of dying people. *Soc Sci Med*. **32**: 943–52.

5 Field D and Copp G (1999) Communication and awareness about dying in the 1990s. *Palliative Med*. **13**: 459–68.

6 General Medical Council (1998) *Good Medical Practice*. General Medical Council, London.

7 Elwyn G, Joshi H, Dare D, Deighan M and Kameen F (2001). Unprepared and anxious about 'breaking bad news': a report of two communication skills workshops for GP registrars. *Educ Gen Pract*. **12**: 34–40.

8 Fletcher C (1980) Listening and talking to patients. *BMJ.* **281**: 994–6.

9 Kaye P (1995) *Breaking Bad News: a ten-step approach.* EPL Publications, Northampton.

10 Fallowfield L (1993) Giving sad and bad news. *Lancet.* **341**: 476–8.

11 Buckman R (2000) Communication in palliative care: a practical guide. In: D Dickson, M Johnson and J Katz (eds) *Death, Dying and Bereavement* (2e). Sage Publications, London.

12 Ptacek JT and Eberhardt TL (1996) Breaking bad news: a review of the literature. *JAMA.* **276**: 496–502.

13 Girgis A and Sanson-Fisher RW (1998) Breaking bad news. 1. Current best advice for clinicians. *Behav Med.* **24**: 53–9.

14 Buckman R and Kason Y (1992) *How to Break Bad News: a guide for health-care professionals.* Papermac, London.

15 Barnett M, Fisher J, Cooke H, Dale J and Irwin C. *Unpublished Report.*

16 Baile W and Buckman R (1998) *Pocket Guide to Communication Skills in Clinical Practice, Including Breaking Bad News.* Cine-Medic Productions Inc., Toronto.

17 Hogbin B and Fallowfield LJ (1989) Getting it taped: the bad news consultation with cancer patients. *Br J Hosp Med.* **41**: 330–33.

18 McHugh P, Lewis S, Ford S *et al.* (1995) The efficacy of audiotapes in promoting psychological well-being in cancer patients: a randomised controlled trial. *Br J Cancer.* **71**: 388–92.

19 Kübler-Ross E (1969) *On Death and Dying.* Macmillan, New York.

20 Kastenbaum R (1991) *Death, Society and Human Experience* (4e). Merrill, New York.

21 Benson J and Britten N (1999) Respecting the autonomy of cancer patients when talking with their families: qualitative analysis of semistructured interviews with patients. *BMJ.* **319**: 293–6.

22 Jolly H (1981) When a child dies. In: H Jolly (ed.) *Book of Child Care* (3e). George Allen & Unwin Ltd, London.

23 Barnes J, Kroll L, Burke O, Lee J, Jones A and Stein A (2000) Qualitative interview study of communication between parents and children about maternal breast cancer. *BMJ.* **321**: 479–82.

24 Nelson E, Sloper P, Charlton A and White D (1994) Children who have a parent with cancer. A pilot study. *J Cancer Educ.* **9**: 30–36.

25 British Medical Association (1995) *Advance Statements About Medical Treatment.* British Medical Association, London.

26 Voltz R, Akabayashi A, Reese C, Ohi G and Sass H (1998) End-of-life decisions and advance directives in palliative care: a cross-cultural survey of patients and health-care professionals. *J Pain Symptom Manage.* **16**: 153–62.

27 Danis M, Garrett J, Harris R and Patrick DL (1994) Stability of choices about life-sustaining treatments. *Ann Intern Med.* **120**: 567–73.

28 Wilks M (2000) Legal issues need clarification. *BMJ.* **321**: 705.

29 Parkes CM (1996) *Bereavement: studies of grief in adult life* (3e). Routledge, London.

30 Stroebe MS and Stroebe W (1993) The mortality of bereavement: a review. In: MS Stroebe, W Stroebe and RO Hansson (eds) *Handbook of Bereavement: theory, research and intervention.* Cambridge University Press, Cambridge.

31 Bowlby J (1980) *Attachment and Loss. Vol. 3. Loss: sadness and depression*. Hogarth Press and Institute of Psychoanalysis, London.

32 Shuchter Z (1993) The course of normal grief. In: MS Stroebe, W Stroebe and RO Hansson (eds) *Handbook of Bereavement: theory, research and intervention*. Cambridge University Press, Cambridge.

33 Woof WR and Carter YH (1997) The grieving adult and the general practitioner: a literature review in two parts. Part 2. *Br J Gen Pract*. **47**: 509–13.

34 Charlton R and Dolman E (1995) Bereavement: a protocol for primary care. *Br J Gen Pract*. **45**: 427–30.

35 Saunderson EM and Ridsdale L (1999) General practitioners' beliefs and attitudes about how to respond to death and bereavement: qualitative study. *BMJ*. **319**: 293–6.

CHAPTER 4

Pain control in palliative care

Carole Anne Tallon

Introduction

This chapter deals with the specific symptom of pain in the primary palliative care setting. When managing pain it is important to know one's enemy, so that one may equip oneself with the knowledge and expertise necessary to alleviate this unpleasant symptom. This requires an understanding of what pain is and why it is present in illnesses such as cancer. It also involves understanding how a person responds to pain on a physical and emotional level, as well as knowing how to assess the pain, recommend appropriate management and address the patient's individual concerns about their pain.

What is pain?

Pain is a personal and individual experience. It has a combination of physical and emotional components, and it consists of what the patient says hurts. This makes the management of pain very challenging both for the patient and for the primary healthcare team.

The definition of pain by the International Association for the Study of Pain describes it as 'an unpleasant sensory and emotional experience associated with actual or potential tissue damage or described in terms of such damage'.[1] So, for example, when a patient says that it feels as if someone is stabbing them with a knife, they are describing the pain in terms of potential damage.

Why do we experience pain?

Pain perception evolved in humans in order to protect the species. It warns us of danger (i.e. actual or potential tissue damage) so that we may take evasive and protective action. For example, when we are burnt by the sun or a hot oven, we know that we need to remove ourselves from the source of the pain in order to prevent further damage. Of course it is not always possible to remove ourselves from the source of pain – for example, when it is caused by a broken bone or the growth of a tumour, pain may continue and often worsen in intensity.

Because of these circumstances, humans also evolved the means of controlling pain – within the nervous system there are natural painkilling peptides called endogenous opioids. Understanding the site and mechanism of action of these peptides has helped us to understand better the nature of pain and also how to develop external means of controlling it.

Pain and the hospice movement

The twentieth-century approach to disease and illness involved aggressive attempts at cure. This was at the expense of developing good symptom control and also at the expense of recognising the patient's personal and emotional needs. In other words, medicine seemed to be failing a large number of patients. Dame Cicely Saunders had observed that dying patients tended to have unmet needs, particularly pain and nausea, but also many other physical and emotional problems. Together with others, she founded a new approach to the management of such patients, which is often thought to represent the birth of the modern hospice movement. The principles of this new approach were to address the patient's symptoms irrespective of the diagnosis and prognosis, and to affirm their lives as being worthy of such effort. Much of Dame Cicely's work involved the use of opiates for the management of cancer-related pain, and recognition of the importance of adequate analgesia.

The scale of the problem

Pain is common in all dying patients. Around 75% of individuals with cancer have at least one source of pain. Some of the pains are due to the cancer itself within the various body tissues, some are due to cancer treatment, and others are due to debility and concurrent disorders. Around 65% of patients dying from other diseases also experience pain. It is known that pain is generally under-treated, yet in the majority of cases it can be successfully relieved.

Box 4.1   The ten commonest pains in cancer patients

- Bone
- Visceral
- Nerve compression
- Soft tissue
- Muscle spasm
- Chronic postoperative pain
- Low back pain
- Constipation
- Oesophagitis
- Capsulitis of the shoulder

How do we feel pain?

We have many pain receptors within our skin, periosteum, arterial walls, joint surfaces and the lining of our cranial vault. Tumours or other damage to these body tissues stimulate many local pain receptors and result in severe pain which can be relatively easy to localise.

Other tissues are only very weakly but diffusely supplied with pain receptors, especially the organs within the body cavities, namely the viscera. We experience pain from visceral organs partly when the source of pain stimulates a diffuse area of pain receptors within those viscera. For example, when an area of the bowel has an occluded blood supply, the ischaemia stimulates a diffuse number of nerve endings to cause pain. The nature of this pain is different to that experienced when surface (or parietal) body parts with many pain receptors are stimulated. This is why patients with cancer sometimes find it difficult to describe or localise their pain. Some viscera, namely the liver parenchyma and the lung alveoli, have almost no pain receptors within them and are in themselves insensitive to pain. However, the liver capsule and bile ducts as well as the bronchi and parietal pleura are extremely sensitive to pain, so tumours within those organs will cause pain when these sensitive components are affected (e.g. by infiltration, swelling or obstruction of a hollow viscus).

What are pain receptors?

Pain receptors are free nerve endings which are activated by noxious stimuli such as pressure (mechanoreceptors), extremes of temperature (thermoreceptors) and chemical substances such as histamine and prostaglandins (chemoreceptors) to produce so-called nociceptive pain. Pain receptors are also called nociceptors. Unlike other sensory receptors, they do not adapt to sustained stimulation but keep on firing signals. This is the reason why pain can become chronic, and it has evolved because of the continued need for the person to remember to protect that area of damage as well as to continue stimulating the endogenous pain control mechanisms.

What carries the signals to the brain?

There are two main types of sensory nerve which carry the signals from the nociceptors, namely the A-delta fibres and the C fibres. The A-delta fibres carry fast acute pain signals, while the C fibres carry the slower chronic pain signals. The nerves synapse in the spinal cord at the level where they enter it, and then other nerve fibres carry the signal up to the brain, where there are synapses in the thalamus and hypothalamus as well as the cerebral cortex. The synapses in the spinal cord and brain are the areas where the opioid receptors are found, so the endogenous opioids exert their action at these points to reduce pain intensity. The same receptors are exploited by exogenous opioids that are prescribed for the patient.

What is the difference between nociceptive and neuropathic pain?

Neuropathic pain differs from nociceptive pain in that the pain signal is not evoked by stimulation of the nociceptors. Neuropathic pain arises when the nerve itself is damaged by compression or infiltration and sends signals of pain to the rest of the nervous system. The damage may affect any nerve within the central or peripheral nervous system. Examples of such damage include invasive or expansive tumour growth, viral infection, or damage following surgery, radiotherapy or chemotherapy, or after events such as a stroke.

Neuropathic pain has a different quality to nociceptive pain. Because the sensory fibres are damaged, the pain will be experienced in an area of numbness. The pain is often described as burning, stabbing, stinging, 'pins and needles' or aching. As well as the numbness, it is sometimes associated with allodynia (abnormal sensation in which a stimulus not usually associated with pain, such as light touch, evokes the pain) or dysaesthesia (an unpleasant sensation in the distribution of the affected nerve). This unpleasant sensation is sometimes described as being like the feeling of insects crawling on the skin, but it is not necessarily painful, and it may be either spontaneous or evoked by various stimuli.

Whereas nociceptive pain responds well to opioids, neuropathic pain is generally only partially responsive. Therefore when treating neuropathic pain other drugs are usually required in addition to opioids.

Assessing the patient's pain

We know that not only is pain common in cancer patients, but also in the 75% of patients who experience pain, on average one-third have one pain, one-third have two pains and one-third have three or more pains. Therefore, it is helpful to find out about the patient's pain or pains during the early stages of management so that treatment can be targeted effectively. Recording this information enables the team to monitor the patient's progress and their response to treatment, as well as providing a means of communicating with the other team members.

Pain assessment tools

Pain history
This includes questions about the site, nature and duration of pain, as well as relieving and exacerbating factors. It also involves finding out about associated symptoms, and how the pain affects the patient's functioning and quality of life, as well as their ideas and concerns about, and expectations of, their pain.

As with all aspects of history taking, listening and empathising, whilst employing one's knowledge of pain to explore the problem thoroughly, will usually lead to accurate deductions which can then form the basis of well-focused management plans in which the patient has confidence.

Examination

This includes a thorough yet focused clinical examination to support the deductions made during the pain history. It not only helps to confirm the cause of the pain or pains, but also elicits information about other aspects of the patient's condition, such as weight loss, nutrition and concurrent medical conditions, as well as functional ability. If the patient agrees to be examined, they almost always find this to be a reassuring and therapeutic experience in itself.

Investigations

These may be necessary if the diagnosis is in doubt or if the results will alter the management (e.g. radiographs for bone pain, serum calcium levels in cases of unexplained abdominal pain).

Body charts

These are pictures of the human body on which the patient can indicate and record the location of their pain(s). The team can annotate the charts with information about the history and physical findings and the likely causes, as well as management to date. If they are kept in the patient's records, these charts can be updated as the care proceeds.

Numerical scales and visual analogue scales

These are one-dimensional instruments for measuring pain intensity or pain relief. With the numerical scale, the patient is asked to give the pain a number according to a described scoring system. Serial scores can then be examined to assess changes in pain. With the visual analogue scale, the patient is asked to give the pain a position on a line, the ends of which denote the extremes of a spectrum ranging from no pain to worst possible pain, or from no pain relief to complete pain relief.

Picture scales

These scales are useful for children or for people with learning disability. The patient is shown a series of pictures, usually faces depicting various emotions ranging from happiness to extreme distress. The patient is then asked to indicate which picture most accurately reflects how their pain makes them feel.

Pain questionnaires and inventories

These are multi-dimensional instruments which question the patient about various parameters relating to the pain, such as pain intensity, mood, pain relief, etc. They use a variety of methods to quantify these variables to provide a scoring system.

With the exception of the history and examination, all of the above assessment tools have limitations in that they only consider certain facets of the patient's pain, and the patient may have difficulties in using them.

Basic principles of successful analgesia

Pain control is not simply about assessing a patient's pain and then prescribing the right combination of drugs. Since we know that pain perception is an individual experience, it follows that its management must be individualised. Moreover, not only is pain a physical experience, but there are many other factors, such as emotions and social circumstances, which also play a major role. Therefore the therapeutic options will include addressing the emotional and social issues and discussing and negotiating with the patient the management plan that suits them best, both physically and emotionally.

This negotiation will involve managing the patient's expectations and setting realistic goals. For example, the patient may lose confidence if, after assessment and initial management, the pain is still present. A good short-term goal might be to aim to obtain a good night's sleep, and then set later goals of being more comfortable during the day.

Options for successful analgesia include a combination of non-drug and drug measures.

Non-drug options for analgesia

It is important to address factors which lower the pain threshold. These include insomnia, anxiety, depression, social isolation and inactivity.

Non-drug options for analgesia include the following:

* physiotherapy and exercise
* transcutaneous electrical nerve stimulation (TENS)
* acupuncture
* cognitive therapy
* radiotherapy
* heat pads
* homeopathic treatments (e.g. aromatherapy).

Drug options for successful analgesia

In order to consider the options, we shall divide pain into two categories:

* opioid-responsive pain
* pain that is partially responsive to opioids.

Opioid-responsive pain: drug options

Management involves each of the following principles:

* by the mouth
* by the clock
* by the ladder.

By the mouth
Encourage use of the oral route for all steps on the ladder unless the patient's condition or preference dictates otherwise.

Alternative routes include rectal, percutaneous endoscopic gastrostromy, transdermal, subcutaneous, intravenous and intrathecal or epidural routes.

By the clock
Cancer pain is continuous and therefore PRN ('as needed') analgesia is not appropriate. Analgesia should be given regularly and prophylactically.

By the ladder
The World Health Organization analgesic ladder[2] is illustrated in Figure 4.1.

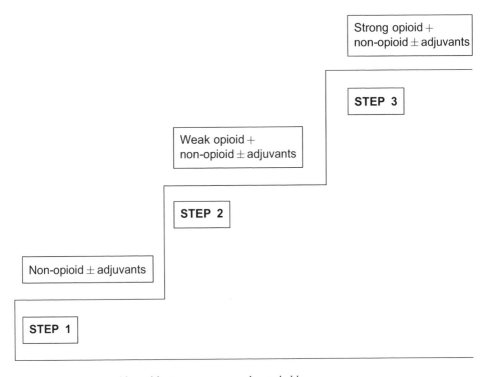

Figure 4.1   The World Health Organization analgesic ladder.

Step 1
If the patient is not on analgesics, start with a simple non-opioid analgesic such as paracetamol or aspirin. Adjuvants may also be used at this stage.

Step 2
If step 1 drugs fail to control the patient's pain, then give an opioid drug for mild to moderate pain (so-called 'weak' opioids) such as codeine, dihydrocodeine, co-dydramol, co-proxamol or tramadol. Note that tramadol is a step 2 *and* a step 3 drug.

Also add non-opioids and adjuvants if necessary. Note that the patient may be taking paracetamol as a co-drug with the opioid.

Step 3

If step 2 drugs do not control the patient's pain, then recommend that they take opioids for moderate to severe pain (so-called 'strong opioids') such as morphine or hydromorphone. Again add non-opioids and adjuvants if necessary.

The above principles apply generally to pain control. However, in patients with severe pain this strategy may be too slow to ensure satisfactory pain control within a short time. In such cases it is necessary to use one's judgement as to whether steps 1 or 2 should be omitted. Cancer pain can be severe and complex, so careful evaluation and assessment together with regular re-evaluation can lead to individualised satisfactory palliation.

What is an opioid?

An opiate is a specific term for a natural or semi-synthetic drug derived from the juice of the opium poppy (e.g. morphine). Opiates have strong analgesic properties as well as many other, mainly unwanted effects.

An opioid means an opiate-like drug, which is a general term describing a natural, semi-synthetic or synthetic drug with morphine-like activity. Opioids act at the same receptors as opiates, and their action is reversed by the morphine antagonist naloxone.

Opioids were initially synthesised in an attempt to reduce the unwanted effects of morphine, such as tolerance and dependence, but most of them share many properties with morphine. Synthetic drugs include diamorphine, methadone, dihydrocodeine and fentanyl.

Box 4.2   Common side-effects of morphine

- *Sedation.* Common at the start of treatment, but wears off after a few days.
- *Nausea and vomiting.* Nausea is very common in the first few days, but vomiting is less so. Can be controlled by giving anti-emetics during the first few days of treatment. Do not forget to review this after a week.
- *Constipation.* This occurs in almost all patients. Give prophylactic laxatives in all patients unless contraindicated.
- *Dry mouth.* This occurs in most patients. Combat with simple measures.
- *Respiratory depression.* This side-effect can be useful for breathlessness in low doses, but in excess it can be potentially problematic.
- *Cough suppression.*
- *Itching.*
- *Myoclonic jerks.*

Choosing the dose
- The right dose of an analgesic is that which relieves the pain.
- If there are constraints due to the pharmacokinetics (e.g. paracetamol, which has a maximum dose of 4 g/24 hours), then move up the ladder.
- There is no advantage in moving from one drug at step 2 to another step 2 drug unless there is a clear increase in dose.

Example
A man with soft-tissue pain from a mediastinal tumour that is not well controlled by taking paracetamol 1 g four times daily (qds) should then move on, for example, to co-codamol 8/500 2 tablets qds.

If there is not enough pain relief, choose a step 2 opioid, such as co-codamol 30/500 2 tablets qds.

If there is not enough pain relief, maximal regular step 2 is considered to be equivalent to morphine (immediate release) 10 mg 4-hourly. Convert to this regime and monitor the pain.

If there is not enough pain relief, there is no maximum dose of morphine while the patient is still experiencing pain, so titrate the dose against the pain. An increase of dose by 30–50% every 2–3 days or sooner is appropriate. For example, on day 2 or 3 increase to 15 mg every 4 hours (an increase of 50%). A double dose at bedtime may avoid the need for the early-morning dose.

The pain should be reassessed daily, and the patient or carer may keep a log of the pain and the analgesia taken.

It is not uncommon for patients to need at least 30 mg morphine 4-hourly (200 mg/24 hours).

Once the patient's pain is stable, maintenance medication has to be decided.

Options for maintenance opioids include the following.

- Continue 4-hourly immediate-release morphine.
- Change to 12-hourly sustained-release morphine.
- Change to 24-hourly sustained-release morphine.
- Change to transdermal fentanyl patch.
- Change to another strong opioid.

The choice will largely depend on what the patient feels will suit their lifestyle best. If using modified-release preparations, ensure that the patient has immediate-release morphine available to take as often as required for episodes of break-through pain. The breakthrough dose is the equivalent 4-hourly morphine dose. If the patient is requiring frequent breakthrough doses, then he or she should be reassessed and may need further analgesia titration.

What are the relative potencies of the various opioids?
It is useful to know about the relative potencies of the various opioids, so that if the patient needs to change from one drug to another, the appropriate dose may be calculated.

Table 4.1 Relative potencies of the different opioids

Analgesic drug	Potency ratio to oral morphine	10 mg oral morphine equivalent (mg)	Duration of action (hours)
Dextromoramide	2	5	2–3
Pethidine PO	1/8	30–60	2–3
Pethidine IM	1/8	75–125	2–3
Codeine	1/12	120	3–6
Dextropropoxyphene	1/10	100	3–6
Hydromorphone	6	2	4–5
Oxycodone	1.5–2	15–20	4–5
Diamorphine	1.5	6	4–6
Tramadol	1/4	40	4–6
Methadone	5–10	3–12	8–12
Fentanyl	150*	Not applicable	72

* To calculate conversion between fentanyl and morphine, *see* Table 4.3.

Patients sometimes need to change drugs in order to titrate the dose (e.g. when moving from a mild opioid to a stronger one) or for the purpose of rotating or 'switching' opioids in order to maximise efficacy while minimising side-effects. The patient may also need to change drugs in order to change the route of administration either for clinical reasons or because of personal preference.

Important points to consider include the following:

- route of administration – some drugs are more potent when given parenterally and others are more potent in oral form than others
- potency ratio with oral morphine (*see* Table 4.1)
- duration of action – a short duration of action makes a drug impractical for managing pain in a palliative care setting (e.g. pethidine)
- individualisation of care – the conversions provide guidelines, but patients may vary in their response to different drugs and therefore the dosage must subsequently be altered
- titration of dose of the new drug – if changing because of increased pain, the equivalent dose of the new drug will not be effective until it is titrated upwards as described earlier. If the drug is being rotated or 'switched' to minimise side-effects, it is usual to reduce the dose of the new drug by one-third without compromising pain control
- seek specialist advice – when uncertain about a drug or its potency, contact the local palliative care team.

How to write a prescription for opioids
Computer-generated prescriptions offer many advantages to the primary care team in terms of time saved, accuracy of prescribing and adherence to recommended

formularies, which in turn may generate cost-savings. However, the prescribing of a drug subject to the Misuse of Drugs Act 1985 (schedule 2 and 3 controlled drugs) requires that the following elements of the prescription be written by hand, in the prescriber's own handwriting and in ink:

- the name and address of the patient
- the name of the drug
- the form and strength of the preparation
- the total quantity of the preparation, or the number of dose units, in both words and figures.
- the dose that the patient should take
- the number of instalments and intervals (where applicable).

Example
- *Mary Jones*
- *16 High Street, Anytown AT7 2CD*
- *morphine oral solution 10 mg/5 mL*
- *supply 200 mL (two hundred)*
- *to take 20 mg every 4 hours.*

Transdermal fentanyl patches

These are reservoirs of the synthetic opioid fentanyl in the form of skin patches. They are suitable for chronic cancer pain and should be considered for patients with opioid-responsive pain that is stable, and as an alternative to morphine.

Table 4.2   Advantages and disadvantages of transdermal fentanyl patches

Advantages	If patient is unable to take morphine If patient is unable to take oral medications Aids compliance If patient prefers non-oral route Less constipation than with morphine
Side-effects	Same as morphine (although constipation and possibly nausea and sedation are less severe) Reversed by naloxone
Contraindications	Acute pain where rapid dose titration is required Sensitivity to fentanyl Sensitivity to silicone adhesive
Cautions	Patients requiring low doses of opioids ($<$60 mg morphine/24 hours) Pyrexia makes rate of absorption unpredictable

Preparations
There are four patch sizes: 25, 50, 75 and 100. Note that if the patient requires a higher dose, an appropriate combination of patches should be calculated.

The number is equivalent to the number of micrograms delivered per hour. The patch should last for 72 hours.

Managing the patient on a fentanyl patch
- After application of the first patch, plasma levels rise for 24 hours and analgesic levels are reached by 6–12 hours. Steady state is reached by the time the patch is replaced (usually 72 hours).
- The patch should be replaced every 3 days at the same time of day.
- Warn the patient that they may have more breakthrough pain than usual in the first 1 to 3 days.
- Immediate-release opioid should be readily available for breakthrough pain (the equivalent 4-hourly morphine dose; *see* Table 4.3).
- Titrate the dose upward in steps of 25 micrograms/hour at each patch change.
- Apply the patch to clean, dry, non-hairy, flat skin.
- Choose a different skin site for each change.
- Reduce laxatives by 50% and titrate according to need.

Table 4.3 Conversion table for oral morphine, transdermal fentanyl and subcutaneous diamorphine

4-hourly oral morphine dose (mg)	24-hourly oral morphine dose (mg)	Fentanyl patch size (micrograms/hour)	24-hourly subcutaneous diamorphine (mg)
5–20	30–130	25	10–40
25–35	140–220	50	50–70
40–50	230–310	75	80–100
55–65	320–400	100	110–130
70–80	410–480	125	140–170
85–95	500–570	150	180–200

How does a patient convert from morphine to fentanyl patches?
- If converting from 4-hourly morphine, the patient should continue regular immediate-release morphine until peak plasma levels are reached (i.e. the first 12–24 hours).
- If converting from 12-hourly modified-release morphine, the patient or the carer should apply the patch at the same time as the final 12-hourly tablet is taken.
- If converting from 24-hourly modified-release morphine, the patch should be applied 12 hours after taking the final 24-hourly capsule.

Syringe drivers
Syringe drivers are small battery-operated infusion pumps designed to deliver the infusion into the subcutaneous tissues.

Two of the commonest pumps in use are the following:

• Graseby MS16 (Blue) set at mm/hour (usually 0.2 mm/hour)
• Graseby MS26 (Green) set at mm/day (usually 48 mm/24 hours).

The volume contained in 48 mm of the syringe (approx 8–9 mL in a 10-mL syringe) will then be that delivered over a period of 24 hours.

Syringe drivers are useful for the following reasons.

• They provide a convenient non-oral route of administration.
• They provide steady plasma concentrations of drug.
• They avoid the need for repeated injections.
• They are light and small enough for the patient to remain ambulant.
• More than one drug can be given in the infusion (seek advice on compatibility, e.g. from specialist palliative care team or pharmacist).

The disadvantages of subcutaneously infused drugs are as follows.

• The patient's needs must be anticipated for the next 24 hours.
• Any increase in the patient's requirements necessitates additional injections until the infusion can be changed.
• People may associate them with imminent death.
• The patient may find them inconvenient or obtrusive.

As with all aspects of palliative medicine and general practice, the key to success is to anticipate and listen to the patient's concerns and to give thorough explanations and reassurances about the options that are chosen.

Indications for a syringe driver
These are as follows:

• oral route not appropriate due to nausea, vomiting, dysphagia, cognitive dysfunction or altered consciousness
• other routes also not feasible (e.g. rectal route impractical due to diarrhoea or tumour site, or transdermal route not practical as patient's requirements are not stable or patient requires other drugs that can be delivered subcutaneously).

Setting up a syringe driver
• Dilute drugs in water for injections using a 10- or 20-mL syringe.
• Set the syringe driver rate to deliver the volume in 24 hours.
• Sufficient volume must be allowed to enable priming of the giving set (including Luer locks at either end).

- Label the syringe with the drug contents, date, patient's identity and the identity of the person administering the infusion.
- Insert a fine-needle-gauge butterfly with long tubing at an angle of 45 degrees into the skin of the chosen site (anterior chest wall, outer upper arm, thigh or abdominal wall are the commonest sites).
- Attach the syringe to the pump, ensuring that the plunger is in contact with the barrel of the syringe.
- Protect the mixture from light using the cover or a holster.

Managing a syringe driver

1   Check the syringe driver regularly for:

- irritation at skin site
- crystallisation of drugs
- light flashing (indicates battery is working)
- volume and rate
- patency of giving-set tubes.

2   Educate the patient and their family and provide on-call contact details.
3   Ensure that breakthrough analgesia is available (if patient's needs increase or the syringe driver fails).
4   Ensure that the patient and their family understand that the boost button is not to be used for breakthrough analgesia. Use of the boost does not provide an adequate dose, and it reduces the overall volume in the pump, so the infusion will not last for 24 hours.

Pain that is partially responsive to opioids: drug options

Non-opioids and adjuvant analgesics

Many pains will only be partially relieved by opioids, so other drugs are used in addition to opioids in order to achieve pain control. Non-opioids can be used on all steps of the analgesic ladder, and are not then replaced by the opioids but used in conjunction with them (*see* Table 4.4).

Paracetamol

This is a drug which acts on a variety of receptors within the nervous system to produce analgesia. Its mode of action is not fully understood, but it is effective in relieving many types of pain. It is appropriate for use on all steps of the analgesic ladder, either by itself or with adjuvants for step 1, or with opioids with or without adjuvants for steps 2 and 3. It is advantageous in that it does not cause gastric irritation, but its disadvantages include its short half-life and the fact that it is not available in modified-release forms.

It is important not to overlook paracetamol as a useful and effective painkiller. The fact that it is available over the counter tends to make people mistakenly regard it as weak and inappropriate for cancer pain.

Table 4.4   Indications for non-opioids and adjuvant analgesics

Class of drug	Indications
Paracetamol	Bone pain Soft tissue pain Muscle spasm pain
Non-steroidal anti-inflammatory drug (NSAID)	Bone pain Soft tissue infiltration Hepatomegaly (stretched liver capsule)
Corticosteroids	Raised intracranial pressure Soft tissue infiltration Nerve compression Hepatomegaly (stretched liver capsule)
Antidepressants Anticonvulsants Anti-arrhythmics	Nerve compression or infiltration

Non-steroidal anti-inflammatory drugs (NSAIDs)

These drugs are of particular benefit when the pain is associated with inflammation, such as soft tissue infiltration or bone metastases. These conditions will naturally be associated with local oedema, which will either exert pressure on the surrounding structures, including nerve fibres, or contain chemicals which will stimulate chemo-nociceptors and so cause pain. This is why NSAIDs can be used for both nociceptive and neuropathic pain.

NSAIDs work by inhibiting the production of cyclo-oxygenase enzyme (COX), which is important for the conversion of arachidonic acid to prostaglandins. There are two forms of COX. COX-1 is constitutive (i.e. present in normal tissues) and COX-2 is inducible (i.e. produced in large quantities when there is inflammation, but normally undetectable). Inhibition of COX-1 is thought to be the main cause of the gastrointestinal side-effects of NSAIDs, whilst inhibition of COX-2 results in anti-inflammatory effects.

Table 4.5   Examples of NSAIDs

Drug	COX selective or non-selective
Ibuprofen	Non-selective
Diclofenac	Non-selective
Naproxen	Non-selective
Diflunisal	Non-selective
Rofecoxib	COX-2 selective
Celecoxib	COX-2 selective

Box 4.3 Points to consider when choosing a non-steroidal anti-inflammatory drug

Side-effects
These vary in severity and frequency. They include gastrointestinal irritation, bleeding and ulceration.
They can also cause renal impairment, so in patients with renal, cardiac or hepatic impairment they must be used with caution.
Patients vary in their tolerance of these drugs. If one NSAID has caused intolerable side-effects, it may be worth cautiously trying another instead.

COX-1 and COX-2 inhibition
NSAIDs vary in their selectivity for inhibition of COX-1 and COX-2. Theoretically, a selective COX-2 inhibitor should improve gastrointestinal tolerance.

Efficacy
This is similar for all NSAIDs, whether a non-selective COX or a selective COX-2 inhibitor.

Safety
NICE guidelines suggest that COX-2 inhibitors are safer for certain patients when being used for long-term treatment of arthritis.[3] We do not yet have data to show whether there is a difference in the safety profile when using them in patients with cancer-related pain.

It is recommended that a gastroprotective drug such as a proton pump inhibitor (PPI) is co-prescribed with NSAIDs in patients who are more likely to be vulnerable to the unwanted effects (e.g. patients aged over 65 years, those on anticoagulants or taking corticosteroids, or those with a history of gastrointestinal bleeding or perforation).[4]

Adjuvant analgesics

These are drugs that are not classed as analgesics because they are used primarily for other indications. They do act as analgesics in some painful conditions, and are therefore useful to combine with other drugs on all steps of the analgesic ladder. Adjuvant analgesics are sometimes called co-analgesics.

Corticosteroids (steroids)

These are useful adjuvants when the pain is due to nerve compression by tumour. It is thought that they work by reducing inflammation and oedema around the tumour. This in turn reduces the pressure on the nerve.

Commonly used steroids are prednisolone and dexamethasone. Dexamethasone is 7.5 times more potent than prednisolone. Therefore 8 mg of dexamethasone is equivalent to approximately 60 mg of prednisolone.

In general, it is thought to be more efficacious to commence with a high dose and then rapidly reduce it with a view to withdrawal or maintenance on the lowest dose possible. Steroids should be administered in the morning to avoid the peak of mental stimulation during the night. There is no benefit in giving steroids more than once a day unless the patient cannot tolerate the number of tablets when they are all administered at once.

Antidepressants

Tricyclic antidepressants (TCAs) are useful for many pains that are only partially opioid responsive, such as neuropathic pain and chronic pain syndromes, and particularly pain that has a constant, burning or aching nature. The most commonly used tricyclic antidepressant is amitriptyline, but other TCAs such as dothiepin, clomipramine, imipramine and lofepramine can all be used, the latter two tending to be less sedative.

Selective serotonin reuptake inhibitors (SSRIs) also act as analgesics, but are less efficacious than the TCAs.

The newer antidepressant mirtazapine, which increases both noradrenaline and serotonin levels, is showing promise as an adjuvant analgesic. This is a noradrenaline and selective serotonin antidepressant (NASSA).

Anticonvulsants

Anticonvulsant drugs such as carbamazepine, sodium valproate and gabapentin are useful adjuvants for neuropathic pains, particularly those with a shooting nature. It is usual to start treatment with a low dose and to titrate upwards depending on how well the patient tolerates the side-effects.

Anti-arrhythmics

Because these drugs act as membrane stabilisers in body tissues, they can act as analgesics by reducing unwanted activity along a nerve. Intravenous lidocaine (Lignocaine) has been shown to reduce neuropathic pain in some patients, and the effect has been sustained by maintaining the patient on oral anti-arrhythmics.

Examples of oral drugs that are used include mexiletine and flecainide. Because these drugs are not commonly used and a cardiac risk may be associated with them, it is advisable to seek advice and assistance from a specialist in palliative medicine or a pain anaesthetist.

Role of the pharmacist

The pharmacist has an important role within the primary care team both as a source of advice and information for patient and primary care team members and in the practical role of dispensing medications or assisting with the preparation of medication for a syringe driver. Input from the pharmacist in palliative care can be pivotal, particularly when the patient's symptoms are being managed with medications. It is helpful if the patient tends to go to the same local pharmacy, so that the pharmacist is involved in the overall care and monitoring of the patient's management and computer records of medicines previously dispensed. In an urban setting the patient may go to a variety of pharmacists and lose this added benefit, but they might opt to select just one pharmacy for better continuity of palliative care.

When analgesia is being titrated or changed in response to the progression of the disease, the process can be made much more efficient and less stressful for both patient and primary care team members if the pharmacist is involved. The pharmacist cannot carry unlimited stocks, so if he or she is informed as soon as possible of changes to the patient's prescription, then suppliers can be contacted immediately to ensure a smooth transition from one drug or dosage to another. In practice it is often the district nurse or Macmillan nurse who contacts the pharmacist about drug changes. Another rate-limiting step for the pharmacist can be the generation of the prescription itself. The primary care team should look at this and other steps in the process in order to streamline the process. Practical solutions include the use of fax and email facilities, and there is potential for the development of intranets within the primary care trust in order to optimise efficient communications and so initiate the generation of a prescription.

Doctrine of double effect

Many people are reluctant to prescribe or consume opioids because they believe that these drugs hasten death. Certainly opioids can cause respiratory depression, and in a frail person this may lead to poor ventilation, which in turn may precipitate a chest infection and possibly death. However, in an individual who is taking opioids regularly and at the right dose to palliate their pain, it is almost unheard of that this would cause respiratory arrest.

The high-profile cases that are reported in the media generally revolve around opioids given to people inappropriately (e.g. if they were previously opioid-naive, not in pain or breathless, or receiving too high a dose for their symptoms). If opioids are prescribed with the sole and sincere intention of palliating symptoms, then the further effect of precipitating a chain of events that lead to death is acceptable in a moral sense. This is called the doctrine of double effect, and it has been tested in our legal system in recent years. The distinction between intended and foreseen events allows the use of measures to relieve suffering even though they carry a significant risk of shortening life (*see* Chapter 12 for further discussion of this issue).

Questions that are commonly asked by patients

Question: **If I continue to take painkillers even though I no longer feel pain, then how do I know if I still need them?**

Answer: Many patients wonder about this. Pain warns us of potential damage to our bodies, but once we know about the pain we try to relieve it. If the pain is due to a chronic cause we know it will still be there. If the painkillers work well then you will not feel pain, and this is a good result. If you wish to check whether the pain is still there at any time it is worth discussing with your doctor or nurse if the painkillers could be reduced by a small amount. If the pain reappears after reducing the dose, we know that the painkillers were working and were at the correct dose. If the pain does not reappear after reducing the dose, then we could reduce it further until the pain does reappear, or until you are no longer on pain-killers, whichever comes first.

Question: **If I keep taking these drugs, won't I get addicted to them?**
Answer: Once the dose of your opioid is correct, so that it deals with your pain, it is unusual for you to need to increase your dose because your body has simply 'got used to it'. This would be called tolerance, and it generally only happens if you take opioids when there is no pain. If the pain changes in some way, then your dose may then need to be changed, but it is not because you are addicted.

   If your pain is relieved by other means so that you no longer need your opioids, you will need to reduce the dose by 25% a day in order to stop taking them, rather than stopping them immediately. This is because the body does develop a physical dependence which is reversible if managed in this way. Psychological dependence is very rare in patients with cancer-related pain.

Question: **If I start taking strong drugs at this stage of my cancer, won't they stop working later on when the pain gets worse?**
Answer: Morphine and other opioids are useful drugs in that they are effective painkillers at whatever dose is found to be right for the pain at that time. If you find that your pain responds to opioids at all, then the only thing which limits the amount of opioid that can be taken is the degree of side-effects.

   The way in which opioids work on the body means that doses can be increased according to the intensity of the pain and still be effective. We know from experience that even if one opioid ceases to be effective or the side-effects are too great once a certain dose is reached, we can switch to a different opioid at a lower dose and the side-effects will decrease. This usually controls the pain or gives us further scope for increasing the dose according to the pain.

Question: **Won't taking morphine make me die sooner?**
Answer: Many people associate morphine with imminent death, and this is because it is often only started quite late in someone's illness. People have mistakenly come to believe that it is the morphine which has caused the death, rather than the illness for which the morphine was prescribed.

   We know that when the dose is calculated correctly, and if the drug is taken appropriately, morphine and other opioids are compatible with a normal lifestyle. Many people take opioids for months or even years with no difficulties.

Question: **I want to stay in control of my senses. Won't this take control away?**
Answer: Many people worry that opioids will make them lose control of their senses or of their life. Opioids do cause the side-effect of feeling drowsy when they are first taken or when the dose has to be increased because the pain is not yet controlled or has increased. This side-effect wears off after a few days in most cases. There is no reason why you should lose control if the drug is working well and is being monitored by your doctor or nurse.

If at any time you feel that you are losing control when taking opioids, you should discuss this with your doctor or nurse so that they can check whether the dose is correct and also whether there are any other reasons for your feeling out of control.

Question: **Can I still drive when I take morphine?**
Answer: It is the responsibility of the driver to ensure that he or she is safe to be in control of a motor vehicle. The use of morphine or other opioids does not prohibit someone from driving. However, when morphine is first being taken or the dose is being increased, it may take a few days for the drowsiness to wear off, so it is sensible not to drive at this time.

By law you are not required to inform your motor insurance company that you are taking opioids, but it may be advisable to let them know in order to avoid any contested claims over this issue in the future.

Your GP is not required to inform the DVLA that you are taking opioids. However, there may be other aspects of your illness which do necessitate informing the DVLA.

Question: **My bowels are fine. Why should I take laxatives with morphine?**
Answer: Morphine always causes some degree of constipation because of the way in which it works when it gets into the bowels. Even if your bowels are working regularly, once you start to take any opioid they will start to work more slowly and become constipated. It is better to take laxatives as an insurance against this than to wait until the constipation sets in. We recommend the use of a stimulant laxative to counteract the slowing effect of morphine.

Conclusion

Pain is a distressing symptom for patients and can be a multifaceted problem. Management of a patient's pain can be both challenging and rewarding for the primary care team. Effective pain control can be achieved in the majority of patients if the team has an understanding of what is causing the pain, knows how to assess it and is familiar with the appropriate application of all of the management options, as well as being able to tailor these to the individual patient.

References

1 International Association for the Study of Pain (1986) Classification of chronic pain. *Pain.* **34 (Supplement 3)**: 51–226.
2 World Health Organization (1996) *Cancer Pain Relief.* World Health Organization, Geneva.
3 National Institute for Clinical Excellence (NICE) (2001) *Health Technology Appraisal Guidance on the Use of Cyclo-Oxygenase (COX) II Selective Inhibitors.* NICE, London.
4 Anon. (2000) Are Rofecoxib and Celecoxib safer NSAIDs? *Drugs Ther Bull.* **38**: 81–6.

Further reading

- Despopoulos A (1991) *Color Atlas of Physiology* (4e). Thieme Medical Publishers, New York.
- Doyle D, Hanks GWC and Macdonald N (eds) (1998) *Oxford Textbook of Palliative Medicine* (2e). Oxford Medical Publications, Oxford.
- Fallon M and O'Neill B (1998) *ABC of Palliative Care.* BMJ Books, London.
- Faull C, Carter Y and Woof R (1998) *Handbook of Palliative Care.* Blackwell Science, Oxford.
- Joishy S (1999) *Palliative Medicine Secrets.* Hanley and Belfus Medical Publishers, Philadelphia, PA.
- Randall F and Downie RS (1996) *Palliative Care Ethics: a good companion.* Oxford University Press, Oxford.
- Stalker N (1999) *Pain Control: an open learning programme for healthcare workers.* Open Learning Foundation. Radcliffe Medical Press, Oxford.
- Twycross R and Wilcock A (2001) *Symptom Management in Advanced Cancer* (3e). Radcliffe Medical Press, Oxford.
- Twycross R, Wilcock A and Thorp S (1998) *Palliative Care Formulary.* Radcliffe Medical Press, Oxford.
- West Midlands Palliative Care Physicians (1997) *Palliative Care: guidelines for the use of drugs in symptom control* (2e). Department of Medicines Management, University of Keele, Keele.

Useful website

Scottish Intercollegiate Guidelines Network (SIGN) and Scottish Cancer Therapy Network (2000) *Control of Pain in Patients with Cancer.* SIGN, Edinburgh; http://www.sign.ac.uk

Acknowledgements

The author would like to thank Ajit Barot, Pharmacy Manager, Southam Pharmacy, Warwickshire and Dr Chantal Meystre, Consultant in Palliative Medicine, Integrated Services Directorate for Palliative Medicine, Warwickshire.

CHAPTER 5

Symptoms other than pain
Tim Deegan

Introduction
Aims of palliative care

A person in their final illness spends most of their time at home. Successful symptom control in palliative care patients presents a particular challenge to the primary healthcare team (PHCT). The goals of palliative care include quality of life, good symptom management, adjustment to the situation and a dignified death. Bearing these in mind, symptom management should provide the following:

- anticipation and prevention
- full evaluation
- adequate time for explanation and information
- full consideration of the ideas and wishes of the patient
- informed consent

Some of these steps are more difficult to achieve in a primary care setting than within a hospice. Untreated symptoms risk the development of secondary problems, such as depression. They also cause distress for the patient's relatives and friends.

A combined team approach

GPs are more confident about dealing with symptoms that can be treated with drugs (e.g. nausea and vomiting). Nurses are more confident about dealing with symptoms that involve nursing care (e.g. bladder and bowel control, or bedsores). Patients are less likely to volunteer symptoms that have a lower likelihood of being successfully treated, and such symptoms may go completely undetected unless specifically asked for.

To provide the best possible care, a combined approach with good communication between team members is needed. The relatively limited time available with the patient must be used to the full, and symptoms and pointers to potential future problems must be actively sought. The latter will involve educating patients and carers with regard to what they need to know (e.g. initially minor symptoms suggesting spinal cord compression).

Strengths of the primary healthcare team

With regard to information giving and attention both to detail and to the individual, the primary healthcare team may be in a stronger position than a hospice. The patient is likely to know their GP and district nurse, and may have done so for many years. They in turn are likely to be aware of the circumstances and surroundings unique to that patient. This all helps when planning care for a person. Known and trusted GPs and nurses are ideally placed to provide the information and explanations necessary for patient and carers. They also have better scope for helping to give the patient the respect, consolation, support and companionship that must form an integral part of his or her care.[1]

Respiratory symptoms

Problematic respiratory symptoms are common in patients with advanced cancer. Many of these patients have other associated diagnoses (e.g. chronic obstructive pulmonary disease, COPD), and the incidence of new problems (e.g. pulmonary embolism) is increased. Three common symptoms will be covered here, namely cough, breathlessness and haemoptysis.

Cough

Cough affects up to 80% of palliative care patients.[2] It may cause breathlessness, fatigue, vomiting, insomnia and rib injury. It often causes pain and may cause fear, especially if accompanied by blood. The cause can usually be determined by history and examination, which should look for associated clinical findings (e.g. presence and nature of sputum, wheeze, breathlessness).

Causes

Table 5.1 Malignant and non-malignant causes of cough

Malignant causes	Non-malignant causes
Airway obstruction, damage or pressure exerted by tumour	Acute and chronic infections
Pleural or pulmonary metastases	Pulmonary oedema
Pneumonitis caused by radiotherapy	Pulmonary embolism
Vocal cord injury or paralysis	COPD (likely in patients with lung cancer)
	Drug-induced (e.g. by ACE inhibitors)
	Gastro-oesophageal reflux
	Aspiration (motor neurone disease, multiple sclerosis, brain metastases)

Treatment

Optimise treatment of non-malignant causes and consider the following.

Productive cough
- Positional changes, especially at night.
- Steam inhalation.
- Saline nebuliser.*
- Physiotherapy.
- Postural drainage.
- Antibiotics.

Non-productive cough
- Positional changes, especially at night.
- Cough-suppressant drugs.

Antibiotics, if not being used in an attempt to cure infection, may still be useful on occasion if they are effective in reducing distressing symptoms. For those who are unable to cough adequately, consider the following:

- subcutaneous (s/c) hyoscine hydrobromide or glycopyrronium to reduce secretions
- suction.

Drugs to suppress cough

Demulcents (medicines intended to soothe coughs by direct action on the throat) sometimes help by stimulating salivation and swallowing. Simple linctus is as good as any other. They need frequent use to be effective.

Opioids are effective in cough suppression. Codeine may be inadequate, and stronger opiates may be needed. This could necessitate careful explanation for both patient and carers. Methadone has been used, especially at night, due to its long half-life, but as it can accumulate to dangerous levels its use is probably best avoided in the community.

Nebulised solutions of local anaesthetics can be used if all else fails. Side-effects include risk of aspiration, odd taste, numbness and bronchoconstriction, for which reason it is recommended that a small test dose should be used first. This might be best carried out under specialist supervision initially.

Dyspnoea (breathlessness)

This symptom affects up to 70% of cancer sufferers in the later stages of the disease.[2] It may be especially severe during the last week of life. What is defined as breathlessness depends very much on the perception of the individual patient, and

---

*Nebulised saline produces larger volumes of more easily expectorated mucus, and is therefore not appropriate for those who cannot get rid of the latter.

varies according to the speed of onset, severity, level of functional upset and state of mind of the patient. These all need to be taken into account during assessment.

Box 5.1 Causes of dyspnoea

Due to malignancy
  Cancer obstructing airway, taking up space of lung, infiltrating lung
  Cachexia and weakness reducing strength of muscles
  Pleural effusion
  Pericardial effusion
  Superior vena caval (SVC) obstruction
  Damage to or pain in the chest wall
  Anaemia
  Diaphragmatic splinting
  Lymphangitis carcinomatosis

Secondary to treatment
  Pneumonitis/fibrosis following chemotherapy or radiotherapy

Non-malignant
  Infection
  Coexisting respiratory or cardiac disease
  Pneumothorax
  Pulmonary embolism
  Psychological causes:

- anxiety
- fear
- anger
- frustration
- isolation
- depression

Assessment

The history should consider the psychological factors present and the impact of breathlessness on the patient and those around him or her. It should note the speed of onset, associated symptoms, severity, history of treatment and non-cancer problems, and level of independence. It should cover what the patient does to deal with the symptom and what the patient and carers feel that it means. Many people fear that they might die during attacks of breathlessness, or are worried that they are at risk of choking to death at such times.

When examining the patient, signs in the chest may not be easy to elicit. Patients may be less mobile, and some may be unable to comply with instructions. It is useful to watch the patient trying to do routine things (e.g. mobilising).

Investigations

Full blood count and chest X-ray are often useful.

The following investigations are sometimes useful:

- ultrasound to determine the nature of effusions – some malignant effusions are a mixture of tumour and loculated fluid and are difficult to drain
- specific investigations (e.g. ventilation/perfusion ratio (V/Q) scan if querying pulmonary embolism).

Treatment

Consider whether the patient will be likely to benefit overall from specific treatments for some conditions.[2]

Table 5.2   Causes of dyspnoea

Cause	*Possible treatments*
SVC obstruction, bronchial obstruction	Specialist consideration of radiotherapy, chemotherapy, stenting
Lymphangitis	Chemotherapy, steroids
Pleural effusion	Drainage, chemotherapy, pleurodesis
Pericardial effusion	Non-steroidal anti-inflammatory drugs (NSAIDs) (e.g. diclofenac, naproxen), steroids; specialist consideration for drainage, surgery
Pulmonary embolism	Anticoagulation, analgesia
Ascites	Drainage
Anaemia	Transfusion
Infection	Antibiotics
Coexisting COPD/asthma	Bronchodilator nebulisers (salbutamol, ipratropium); these are often useful in patients with primary or secondary lung cancers who experience breathlessness
Coexisting cardiac failure	Diuretics, ACE inhibitors

Non-pharmacological treatment of the symptom
Arrangements in home and individual rooms

The patient may have to reconsider which leisure activities they wish to pursue. Help the patient to consider changes to or extra help from carers with activities of daily living. Reorganisation of house and sleeping arrangements may be useful. Attention to positioning in bed and chairs can be helpful. Increased ventilation with open windows or a fan to provide a gentle stream of air is beneficial.

Explanation and support

The patient is likely to need help to come to terms with their new limitations. The disability caused by shortness of breath or weakness, and the extra time which has to be set aside by the patient to complete simple tasks such as dressing, can cause depression, anxiety and anger. It should be explained to the patient what is causing the dyspnoea, to help to allay their fears. Some therapists can teach breathing techniques and relaxation exercises, which are very often helpful. Complementary therapies may also be helpful with this symptom.

Pharmacological treatment of the symptom
Opioids

In palliative care the opioids used include some weaker ones (e.g. codeine) and a range of stronger ones. The two main strong opioids are morphine and diamorphine. In the opioid-naive (i.e. those who are not already taking regular doses of an opioid or who have only ever used smaller doses of weak opioids), small doses of morphine administered orally may be adequate to relieve breathlessness. Try starting at 2.5 mg morphine qds (four times a day) + 5 mg at night.

This can be converted to a subcutaneous regime of 5–7.5 mg diamorphine over 24 hours for those who are unable to swallow.

For patients who are on opioids, consider increasing the dose by one step and observe whether there is any benefit or whether any side-effects occur. Make sure that any analgesia regime is also giving adequate control of pain.

Benzodiazepines

These drugs are useful when anxiety and panic cause or complicate breathlessness.

Diazepam is the best choice to begin with, at 2 mg/8 hours PO (by mouth).

Lorazepam has a relatively rapid onset of action and can be given sublingually at a dose of 0.5–2 mg. It can therefore be a useful choice on an as-required basis.

Oxygen

Oxygen should be helpful for severely hypoxic patients, and it may be used in others for a set trial period. However, in most patients it may produce more relief by causing airflow and by giving psychological reassurance. Anxious patients find it stressful to be separated from their mask, which may itself act as a barrier to communication. If it is appropriate and useful at home, oxygen concentrators are easier to use than cylinders, which are heavy and bulky. Nasal prongs are convenient and create less of a barrier than a mask.

Opioids and anxiolytics are useful for controlling breathlessness and agitation in the terminal phase of life (*see* page 90).

Haemoptysis

This is the production of blood from somewhere in the respiratory tract, whether higher up in the larynx or from some deeper source. This symptom frightens both patients and carers, and it occurs in up to 30% of patients with carcinoma of the lung.[3]

Factors other than cancer may cause or contribute to haemoptysis. The commonest alternative causes are infection and pulmonary embolism. Also consider whether a clotting disorder or low platelet count may be present (e.g. in the presence of liver metastases, bone-marrow infiltration or after chemotherapy).

Treatment

Radiotherapy is very useful in cases where the bleeding is likely to have come from one or a few specific tumours. It is usually effective and can be repeated in future if necessary.

Drug treatment

Consider stopping NSAIDs and anticoagulants, and try the following instead:

- tranexamic acid 500 mg four times a day
  or
- ethamsylate 500 mg four times a day.

Massive fatal haemoptysis

This is dealt with in Chapter 7 on emergencies.

Gastrointestinal symptoms

Anorexia

This can be defined as loss of or absence of appetite for food, despite the need for nutrition. It is a very common symptom in palliative care, and has been shown to be present in 80% of patients during the last year of life.[4] For patients, it may cause a degree of social isolation if they are unable to take part in meals with those close to them. Carers frequently worry that failure to eat means that the patient has given up. They also worry that the patient might starve to death. There is a risk that they will insistently try to persuade the patient to eat when he or she cannot do so.

Causes

These include the following:

1 pain
2 physical problems with feeding oneself
3 treatments:

- chemotherapy and/or radiotherapy
- antibiotics
- SSRI antidepressants (e.g. paroxetine, fluoxetine)
- opioids

4 any cause of nausea/vomiting
5 gastrointestinal problems (e.g. tumour, infection, mouth problems)
6 anorexia–cachexia. Some tumours provoke the release of chemicals called cytokines, which are involved in immune responses. Sometimes these alter the metabolism of the body, resulting in muscle breakdown. Studies have shown that this can begin to happen when the tumour is still very small. Poor appetite is commonly a feature, but is not primarily responsible for the weight loss. This is unlikely to be understood by relatives and carers, who often think that the patient is wasting solely because they cannot eat
7 changes in the sensation of taste
8 fatigue – this has numerous causes in advanced cancer, and is frequently itself the cause of poor appetite
9 psychological causes – fear, anxiety and depression are all common causes of anorexia.

Treatment

1 Address causes that can be treated.
2 Arrange referral to a specialist dietitian. This can help with dietary requirements, feeding techniques and use of appropriate supplements (of which there are many) for the individual.
3 Noting patient preferences, careful and skilled use of seasonings and flavourings, and care with the visual presentation of food can all be effective in helping to overcome anorexia.
4 Provide support for the patient and their family, including an explanation of the cause of anorexia. Carers may need help in understanding and accepting that the patient needs less nutrition if they are immobile, and that 'feeding them up' will not improve the prognosis or reverse cachexia. They may also not understand that eating itself may be quite tiring for the patient.
5 Drugs:

- dexamethasone 2–4 mg once a day. Sometimes the improvement is only temporary and disappears after about 2 weeks
- megestrol 80–160 mg once a day (some authorities advocate higher doses)
- metoclopramide 10–20 mg three times a day
- cyproheptadine – this is a weak stimulant of appetite.

6   Alcoholic drinks may be favoured by some patients as helping to improve their appetite. However, ethanol itself does not stimulate appetite.

Total parenteral nutrition (TPN) is rarely indicated in palliative care. It is not without complications, and it necessitates a very intensive level of monitoring, with daily blood tests, etc. It will not reverse the cachexia of advanced cancer. It is important that this is explained to the patient and their carers.

Oral symptoms

Traditionally not as much attention is given to problems arising in the mouth in palliative care as to symptoms such as pain. However, while not denying the significance of other symptoms, patients almost invariably attach a high degree of importance to good oral function and comfort. Mouth problems can make eating and talking difficult, and this can isolate the patient socially and cause problems with nutrition.

As patients become weaker and more debilitated, they are at increased risk of mouth problems and they also become less capable of preventing these problems themselves. Frequent and regular help with oral hygiene becomes essential. Nurses can teach the necessary techniques to the patient's family and carers.

In patients with advanced cancer, two specific situations are common:

- dry mouth
- oral thrush.

Dry mouth

This may be caused by any of the following:

- opioids
- beta-blockers
- diuretics
- anticonvulsants (which may be used for neuropathic pains)
- anticholinergic drugs (e.g. hyoscine butylbromide).

In addition, the following factors predispose to dry mouth, infection and other problems:

- immune compromise
- increasing age
- chemotherapy or local radiotherapy
- smoking
- poor oral hygiene
- reduced salivation.

Fungal infections

These usually present with the following symptoms:

* soreness of mouth
* distorted or reduced sensation of taste
* dysphagia.

On examination, you may see the following:

* white plaques
* smooth redness of tongue and/or mucous membranes
* inflammation in the corners of the mouth.

Most fungal infections are due to *Candida albicans*, which is usually sensitive to nystatin and itraconazoles. However, some are due to other species of *Candida* which are often resistant to nystatin and sometimes to other treatments, too.

Treatment

The key to preventing problems is regular mouth care. This may be necessary as often as every 2 hours in patients who are debilitated or at high risk of problems.[5] Attention must be paid to the lips, tongue, gums, teeth and mucous membranes. *Note*: do not forget to include dentures.

For dry mouth, try the following:

* bicarbonate mouthwashes to try to prevent fungal infections
* stimulation of saliva with lemon juice[3]
* replacement of saliva with artificial sprays such as glandosane. However, a recent small study suggested that sugar-free chewing gum might be more useful in almost every respect.[5] Neither of these has the antiseptic properties of saliva
* cubes or juice of pineapple if there is debris in the mouth, as these contain an enzyme that may help to clear it. Pineapple and lemon are likely to cause pain if the mouth is already very sore, cracked or ulcerated
* effervescent vitamin C tablets placed on the tongue are said to help with cleaning, although there is not much evidence for this.

Treatment of fungal infections is probably best achieved with the following:

* fluconazole 50 mg once a day for 1 week – this is usually very effective
* nystatin administered orally can be used instead, but needs to be given several times a day and must be applied very thoroughly throughout the mouth if it is to work properly.

Other causes of soreness

These include various causes of ulceration, most of which will be aphthous ulcers. The latter can be treated with the following:

* benzydamine mouthwashes
* chlorhexidine mouthwashes are helpful in some cases
* adcortyl in Orabase applied to the ulcers twice a day for 1 week.

Some of them may be herpes or zoster lesions. If these are suspected, they should be treated with a course of oral antivirals. There is no good evidence that topical antivirals are effective.

Hiccup

This apparently minor symptom can be debilitating if it is intractable, and it can cause insomnia and fatigue. Tumours in the abdomen can cause hiccup, particularly if they irritate the vagus or phrenic nerves. Gastric distension, tumours close to the diaphragm and intracranial tumours may also cause hiccup.

This symptom can be difficult to treat.

* Try holding iced water in the oropharynx (right at the back of the mouth).
* If the symptom is thought to be due to gastric distension, try giving asilone 10–20 mL before meals and at bedtime.

Also try the following:

* haloperidol (small dose)
* metoclopramide 10 mg three times a day
* baclofen 5–10 mg twice a day
* domperidone 10–20 mg three times a day
* dexamethasone 4 mg once a day
* modified-release nifedipine 10–20 mg twice a day – check blood pressure before and after starting this
* sodium valproate may be used if the cause lies in the central nervous system.

Nausea and vomiting

There is a high incidence of both nausea and vomiting in patients with advanced cancer. Around 40% of patients will experience nausea, and 30% will also suffer from vomiting.

The causes are often multifactorial, and these symptoms affect patients with many different types of cancer. The disease, treatments and related psychological factors may all play a part. Intractable vomiting causes carers to feel helpless and gives rise to feelings of isolation and shame in patients. Furthermore, because the gastrointestinal tract is seen as important in sustaining life, patients and carers regard its malfunction as a sign of serious illness or problems.[3]

The history should note the pattern and speed of onset. It should include the nature of vomit (i.e. whether faeculent, bloody, bilious or containing undigested food). It should also note bowel habit and indicators of raised intracranial pressure (ICP). In addition, drug history with any recent changes must be covered.

A full abdominal examination is needed, and signs of raised ICP must be checked for.

Before treating the patient, consider factors such as the following:

- anxiety
- pain
- smells in the vicinity of the patient
- biochemical status (urea, sodium and calcium levels).

The choice of treatment will depend on the cause. Around 30% of palliative care patients with nausea and vomiting will require two anti-emetics given concurrently.[6] There is a less than complete understanding of many of the possible combinations, but some are relatively commonly used and appear to work well. Consult your specialist if you are unsure about this.

Causes

Gastric stasis
This may be caused by any of the following:

1   drugs:

- tricyclic antidepressants (e.g. amitriptyline, dothiepin)
- neuroleptics
- opioids
- anticholinergics

2   ascites
3   tumour infiltration
4   gastritis:

- steroids
- NSAIDs
- radiotherapy
- stress

5   poor functioning of the autonomic nerves that control gut peristalsis. The nausea is often well relieved after vomiting.

Treatment

Causes should be treated wherever possible. For example, consideration should be given to drainage of ascites.

Drugs that can be used to treat gastric stasis include the following:

- metoclopramide 5–20 mg three times a day by mouth or 15–60 mg/24 hours subcutaneously may help nausea while simultaneously improving gastric emptying
- proton pump inhibitors (e.g. omeprazole) are useful for decreasing the amount of gastric secretions produced. Some of these are available in dispersible forms, which may be better absorbed than a tablet in the circumstances
- dexamethasone 8–16 mg once a day may be useful
- hyoscine butylbromide 60 mg/24 hours subcutaneously will decrease secretions but worsens stasis. The oral form of this drug is poorly absorbed.

Gastrointestinal obstruction

In some patients, problems with delayed gastric emptying are either a prelude to or part of a more problematic picture of full obstruction. This is most commonly seen with tumours of the ovary and bowel. However, many other tumours may cause gastrointestinal obstruction.

The usual features are as follows:

- vomiting – usually large volumes, and tending to contain undigested food if obstruction is higher up the gastrointestinal tract, or to be faeculent in nature if obstruction is lower down
- absolute constipation – no passage of faeces or flatus
- abdominal distension – may be less than expected if tumour in the abdomen is causing multiple adhesions
- abdominal pain, usually colicky exacerbations with a constant background pain
- nausea often relieved by vomiting
- normally 'tinkling' bowel sounds are characteristic. However, little may be heard, especially if the peritoneum is infiltrated with or covered by tumour. This may also make palpation of the abdomen less informative than usual.

Obstruction often presents more subtly or insidiously in patients with advanced cancer than is usually the case in other situations.

Treatment

First consider whether other factors are responsible, including the following:

- drugs
- constipation – optimise bowel care
- biochemical imbalances (calcium, potassium)
- unrelated conditions.

In some patients a gastrostomy will allow them to swallow food and fluids while at the same time relieving nausea and vomiting.

For nausea, consider using the following:

• metoclopramide 30–60 mg/24 hours subcutaneously – this is best avoided if there is much bowel activity and colic is a feature, as it is likely to increase it
• haloperidol 2.5–15 mg/24 hours subcutaneously (start at a low dose and work upward if necessary)
• cyclizine 50–150 mg/24 hours subcutaneously
• cyclizine and haloperidol can be combined and do not antagonise each other.

Also consider the following:

• dexamethasone 6–12 mg/24 hours – this can help to relieve pyloric sphincter obstruction; it is unclear whether it increases the likelihood of resolution otherwise
• hyoscine butylbromide 60 mg/24 hours subcutaneously – this helps to relieve colic and reduces secretions. The dose can be increased above this level, and some authorities suggest up to 200 mg/24 hours.
• octreotide 300–1200 micrograms/24 hours subcutaneously – this is more expensive but may succeed in reducing secretion volume when other drugs fail
• omeprazole or a similar drug taken by mouth can reduce the volume of gastric secretions.

In some cases, nasogastric drainage is used to help to prevent vomiting. However, the nasogastric tubes increase secretions by causing irritation. They also make oral administration of liquids or medicines more difficult, and are prone to causing sores and irritation in the nose. In addition, they may be periodically vomited up if the problem persists. Usually it is best to reduce nausea and vomiting to a level that is acceptable to the patient by other means if possible.

Chemical causes
Drugs that may cause nausea and vomiting include the following:

• opioids
• SSRIs
• NSAIDs
• anticonvulsants (they may well be being used for neuropathic pain)
• chemotherapy – some of these drugs cause relatively minor problems, while others can cause very severe nausea that is unrelieved by vomiting.

Metabolic causes include the following:

• hypokalaemia
• hypercalcaemia

- uraemia
- liver failure.

Toxic causes include the following:

- infection
- tumour.

Treatment
Examine the drug regimen.
   Drugs that may be used include the following:

- haloperidol 2.5–15 mg subcutaneously (see comment above) or equivalent oral dose
- metoclopramide 5–20 mg PO three times a day or 15–60 mg/24 hours subcutaneously
- methotrimeprazine 12.5–50 mg PO once a day or 6.25–25 mg/24 hours subcutaneously
- serotonin (5HT$_3$) receptor antagonists for chemotherapy (e.g. ondansetron).

Methotrimeprazine is a potent anti-emetic with several pathways of action. It can be given once a day only if used orally or as subcutaneous injections. However, it can also be very sedating at higher doses. This can be a problem either in making patients too drowsy or, for example, in making them unsteady of gait. Subcutaneous doses of this drug are half of the oral equivalent.
   Remember that about 30% of patients on opioids need an anti-emetic, but that in many such cases, if this nausea is mild it is likely to disappear after a few days on the opioid.

Stretching and irritation of visceral peritoneum
This may be caused by:

- liver metastases and other tumours
- constipation
- gastrointestinal obstruction
- ureteric obstruction.

Pain is often a prominent feature in this situation. In addition to treating causes and using anti-emetics, consider giving dexamethasone, up to 16 mg/24 hours, as this may reduce the effective bulk of tumours by decreasing the oedema (swelling) surrounding them. This is often helpful with liver metastases, for example.

Raised intracranial pressure

This is often caused by brain metastases. Nausea and vomiting are typically worse after lying down, and are accompanied by headaches and possibly drowsiness. Neurological signs, including papilloedema, need not be present.

Again, consider the use of dexamethasone at up to 16 mg/24 hours.

Use the following as a general guide.

1   Oral medications are useful for anticipating and preventing nausea:

  • cyclizine 50 mg three times a day
  • metoclopramide 5–20 mg three times a day
  • haloperidol 1.5–3 mg at night.

2   In established nausea, even if vomiting is absent, gastric stasis occurs and oral medications become much less effective. Subcutaneous injections are then useful for dealing with the immediate situation:

  • cyclizine 50 mg
  • prochlorperazine 12.5 mg
  • metoclopramide 10 mg.

3   Rectal preparations can also be useful in cases of established nausea and vomiting:

  • cyclizine 50 mg three times a day
  • prochlorperazine 50 mg three times a day
  • domperidone 30–60 mg three times a day.

Constipation

This is a common symptom in palliative care patients. The aim in most cases should be to anticipate and prevent it. Laxatives should normally be routinely prescribed at the same time as any moderate or strong opioids.[3] Often patients will require a softener and a stimulant.

Causes

The commonest causes of constipation are as follows:

• poor diet
• poor intake of fluids
• immobility and weakness
• opioids
• tricyclic antidepressants
• hyoscine
• anticonvulsants
• phenothiazines.

Treatment

Laxatives

Table 5.3   Different types of laxative

Type	Medication	Comments
Softeners	Lactulose 10–30 mL bd tds	This is not to everyone's taste. Possible side-effects include wind, bloating and abdominal discomfort
	Docusate 100 mg tds	This is also a mild stimulant
Bulking agents	Ispaghula, Fybogel	These are not useful for opioid-based constipation. They are rarely used in palliative care. However, they may be useful for thickening purposes for ileostomies
Stimulants	Senna, tablets 1 nocte – 4 bd or 5–20 mL bd Bisacodyl 10 mg nocte Codanthrusate, up to 12 capsules bd* Codanthramer 5–20 mL bd*	* These may turn the urine red, and can also cause perianal irritation. Caution should be exercised in bed-bound patients
	Picosulphate 5–10 mL bd	This is a strong stimulant
Suppositories	Glycerine	A softener and mild stimulant
	Bisacodyl	A stronger stimulant that acts fairly rapidly
Enemas	Citrate	Slightly stronger than suppositories
	Arachis oil	A softener. Requires retention by the patient to be effective
	Phosphate	A stimulant

Neurological and other symptoms

Confusion

Confusion is common in palliative care patients. It is one of the most difficult symptoms to cope with in the community, and in many instances hospice or hospital admission will be needed for investigation/treatment or nursing care, or both.

Causes

Drugs that may cause confusion include the following:

- opioids
- benzodiazepines

- antidepressants
- anticonvulsants
- steroids
- histamine (H_2) receptor blockers (e.g. cimetidine, ranitidine)
- anticholinergics (e.g. hyoscine)
- withdrawal from alcohol, benzodiazepines or opioids.

Other causes include the following:

- urinary retention
- constipation
- brain metastases
- infections (chest and urinary tract are particularly common)
- biochemical imbalance of electrolytes
- metabolic − the onset of renal failure or liver failure often reduces the capacity to metabolise or excrete drugs. This may mean that drug doses which were previously appropriate suddenly cause drug concentrations to rise to toxic levels
- hypoxia
- internal haemorrhages (cerebral or gastrointestinal).

Treatment of the symptom
- Try to create a well-lit, quiet environment. Avoid crowding the patient.
- Maintain a rota of familiar and trusted carers.
- Be careful to explain what is going on at all times.
- Remind the patient of recent events.
- Explain that the confusion is due to the illness and that the patient is not 'going mad'.
- Support the family.
- Monitor the patient's mental state.

Insomnia

Insomnia in palliative care has many causes. It is likely to lead to fatigue, which may cause or exacerbate many other problems. If insomnia is regular and intractable it is very distressing to the patient.

Causes
These may include any of the following:

1 daytime drowsiness and napping. This may be expected, as patients become weaker and more tired. However, in some cases it may disrupt night-time sleeping patterns. This is more likely if it is caused by medication
2 disturbing thoughts and unresolved issues
3 nightmares
4 fear of going to sleep − some patients are afraid of dying in their sleep

5   other anxieties
6   depression
7   pain and cramps
8   sweating and flushes
9   breathlessness
10   continence problems
11   drugs – an important cause:

- steroids – dexamethasone is best given either as one dose in the morning or as two doses, in the morning and at midday. Late doses are likely to cause insomnia
- diuretics, especially if given later in the day!
- caffeine – check tea and coffee drinking habits
- some beta-blockers cause vivid and disturbing dreams
- theophyllines
- sympathomimetics.

Treatment
1   Address the treatable causes outlined so far.
2   Discuss the use of treatments with the patient:

- hypnotics – useful in most cases. Half-lives vary widely both between drugs and between individual patients. Care is needed not to cause drowsiness in the morning
- chlorpromazine 10–50 mg at night. This reduces agitation. Half-life is about 4 hours
- amitriptyline 25–100 mg at night. This is sedating and antidepressant. However, the antidepressant effects only begin at higher doses, probably about 100 mg/24 hours or higher
- chloral hydrate
- quinine sulphate 200 mg at night is useful for leg cramps. Care is needed because it is toxic in overdose.

Table 5.4   Typical half-lives of hypnotics

Hypnotic	Typical half-life (hours)
Zaleplon	1
Zolpidem	2.5
Zopiclone	5
Temazepam	8
Lormetazepam	10
Loprazolam	12
Nitrazepam	25
Flunitrazepam	35
Flurazepam	70

Symptoms in the terminal phase
Agitation and restlessness

The common physical (and often treatable) causes include the following:

- full rectum
- full bladder
- pain
- breathlessness
- nausea.

Other potential common causes include the following:

- anxiety
- fear and distress
- frustration
- outstanding problems – unresolved problems/issues in relationships can cause marked distress and agitation.

Do not forget the following:

1 biochemical causes (liver or kidney failure; calcium, potassium and glucose levels)
2 drugs:

- opioids
- benzodiazepines (e.g. temazepam)
- hyoscine (often used to dry secretions)
- steroids
- anticonvulsants.

Treatment of specific causes should be followed by support for the patient and those close to them. Then consider using the following:

- midazolam 10–60 mg/24 hours subcutaneously
- methotrimeprazine 12.5–200 mg/24 hours subcutaneously – also effective for nausea
- haloperidol 1.5–30 mg/24 hours subcutaneously.

As with pain control, either start at the lowest doses or, if the patient is already on the drug, calculate a 24-hour dose based on requirements over the last 24 hours. Midazolam has a half-life of 4 hours. Therefore the breakthrough dose required is one-sixth of the calculated 24-hour requirement, in the same way as is calculated for opioids in pain control. Upward adjustment of the dosage is usually done in the same way, too (i.e. by addition of about 30% of the current dose). Methotrimeprazine and haloperidol have considerably longer half-lives.

Muscular spasms (myoclonus)

Causes
These include the following:

- biochemical and metabolic disturbances
- drugs (particularly opioids at higher doses).

These are potentially a prelude to seizures. Treat by addressing causes, and then try the following:

- midazolam – consider beginning subcutaneous infusion or increasing by one step
- phenobarbitone 400–800 mg/24 hours subcutaneously
- clonazepam 1–8 mg orally or 0.5–5 mg subcutaneously, per 24 hours.

Picking at the sheets

This is sometimes due to agitation, and it is thought that it may occasionally be due to hallucinations. Try haloperidol 5–10 mg/24 hours subcutaneously.

Noisy (bubbly) breathing

This occurs when the patient is too weak or drowsy to swallow their oral and respiratory secretions. The patient may well be oblivious to it, but carers are often very distressed by this symptom.
Consider the following:

- patient positioning changes
- gentle physiotherapy
- mouth care, possibly including gentle suction
- giving reassurance to those around the patient
- hyoscine 0.6–2.4 mg/24 hours subcutaneously or in the form of patches (0.5 mg/72 hours)
- glycopyrrhonium 0.8 mg/24 hours subcutaneously.

Skin symptoms
Itching

This is a common problem in patients with advanced cancer. The most frequent causes include the following:

- haematological malignancies
- cholestatic jaundice

- biochemical causes (high blood urea level)
- drugs, especially opioids
- advanced cancer.

Treatment
1   Hot and 'stuffy' environments should be avoided.
2   Frequent application of gentle, hypoallergenic soaps and good moisturisers can be helpful.
3   NSAIDs are often effective for itching that is caused by tumour infiltration.[3]
4   Antihistamines:

- loratadine 10 mg once a day – less sedating than the older drugs. Some authorities suggest that the beneficial effect is also reduced
- chlorpheniramine 4 mg four times a day is more sedating.

Sweating

Causes include the following:

- infection
- chemotherapy
- anxiety.

Address the causes. Then try:

- paracetamol 1 g four times a day
- NSAIDs.

Appendix
Syringe drivers

Syringe drivers are frequently used in palliative care to infuse drugs subcutaneously at a steady rate over 24 hours. There are numerous references above to drugs being given in this way (e.g. methotrimeprazine 12.5 mg/24 hours subcutaneously).

Typically the driver is a box about $15 \times 7 \times 1$ cm in size that contains a small electronically controlled motor, a space for a 10-mL syringe to be clipped in and a protective plastic cover to prevent accidental interference. The motor slowly advances the plunger over a set period of time, thereby delivering the contents of the syringe.

The contents are usually infused under the skin of the chest, abdominal wall or thigh via a butterfly needle that is held in place by a protective adhesive patch. In the above case, 12.5 mg of methotrimeprazine would be dissolved in 10 mL of water and set to infuse over 24 hours.

It takes up to 3 hours for the contents of a syringe driver to start becoming effective when first sited. Therefore the patient may need to have the drug administered by some other means to cover this period.

Advantages
- Syringe drivers allow the patient to remain mobile.
- They administer a constant dose of drug.
- They avoid the need for repeated injections, which are particularly unpleasant for cachectic patients.
- In the community, they are much more likely to be compatible with the amount of nurse and doctor time that is available per patient than, for example, are 4-hourly injections.

Disadvantages
- Syringe drivers may need renewing early if the dose of medication required by the patient is changing. Renewing the syringe is safer than altering the rate of infusion, and is the usual method of alteration (e.g. adhering to a constant infusion rate of 10 mL/24 hours). This helps to avoid calculation errors, and is likely to be the only method of adjustment if two or three drugs are being used simultaneously. However, it does waste more drugs and therefore is more expensive.
- There are certain drug combinations that do not mix well in syringe drivers, as one of the drugs can cause the other to precipitate out of solution. Some drugs, notably NSAIDs, are best dissolved in saline.[3]
- Driver sites require regular observation by carers to ensure that they are not becoming inflamed. Some drugs are more likely to cause inflammation than others (e.g. cyclizine is much more likely to cause inflammation than is diamorphine).
- Patients and especially carers sometimes view syringe drivers as being the 'beginning of the end' or indicating that death is imminent. Some people believe that they are only used to sedate dying patients. This, together with the bad press that diamorphine has received in recent years, means that the use of syringe drivers will always need especially careful discussion with the patient and their carers.

More detailed discussion of the use of syringe drivers can be found in the references listed in the Further Reading section.

References

1 Grande GE, Barclay SIG and Todd CJ (1997) Difficulty of symptom control and general practitioners' knowledge of patients' symptoms. *Palliative Med.* **11**: 399–406.
2 Rawlinson F (2000) Dyspnoea and cough. *Eur J Palliative Care.* **7**: 161–4.
3 Faull C, Carter Y and Woof R (eds) (1998) *Handbook of Palliative Care.* Blackwell Science, London.

4 Rimmer T (1998) Treating the anorexia of cancer. *Eur J Palliative Care.* **5**: 179–81.
5 Davies AN (2000) A comparison of artificial saliva and chewing gum in the management of xerostomia in patients with advanced cancer. *Palliative Med.* **14**: 197–203.
6 Twycross R (1995) *Symptom Management in Advanced Cancer.* Radcliffe Medical Press, Oxford.

Further reading

More detailed advice on treatment of the above symptoms as well as those not covered in this chapter may be found in the following two excellent texts.

- Faull C, Carter Y and Woof R (eds) (1998) *Handbook of Palliative Care.* Blackwell Science, London.
- Twycross R and Wilcock A (2001) *Symptom Management in Advanced Cancer* (3e). Radcliffe Medical Press, Oxford.

These are widely available via medical publishers or at your local district general hospital medical library.

Glossary of terms

ACE inhibitors A family of drugs that block angiotensin-converting enzyme and are used to reduce high blood pressure and to treat heart failure. These drugs are also often prescribed long term for patients who have had a heart attack, and for many diabetic patients. Examples include ramipril, perindopril and lisinopril.
bd Twice a day.
Cachexia (adj. **cachectic**) Wasting, especially of the muscles, associated with advanced cancer.
COPD (**chronic obstructive pulmonary disease**) Known in the past as chronic bronchitis or chronic obstructive airways disease (COAD). A disease often caused by smoking, in which largely irreversible changes occur in the airways to the lungs, resulting in progressively more severe shortness of breath.
H_2-blockers A family of drugs used to reduce gastric acid production. Examples include ranitidine and cimetidine.
$5HT_3$-antagonists Powerful and very expensive drugs used to treat intractable nausea and vomiting when all else fails.
od Once a day.
Opioid Any painkilling drug that acts on the same receptors in the central nervous system as does morphine.
Phenothiazines A large group of drugs used to treat psychoses, which also have other effects (e.g. in the treatment of nausea). Members of this group include chlorpromazine, methotrimeprazine, thioridazine and prochlorperazine.
po Given by mouth.
prn As required.

qds Four times a day.

s/c Subcutaneous (i.e. injected directly underneath the skin).

SSRI (selective serotonin reuptake inhibitor) A type of antidepressant. Examples include fluoxetine (Prozac) and paroxetine (Seroxat).

TCA (tricyclic antidepressant) An older family of antidepressant drugs, also useful for treating other conditions.

tds Three times a day.

Acknowledgements

The author wishes to thank the Information Service Departments of St Christopher's Hospice, Sydenham, London and the Bristol Cancer Care Centre, for providing information, and Dr Sarah Shannon for providing very necessary encouragement to write this chapter.

CHAPTER 6

Complementary therapies in palliative care

Tim Deegan

What is meant by complementary therapies?

Complementary or alternative therapies are used frequently in palliative care to complement and improve symptom control. Most complementary therapies follow a philosophy that is ideally suited to palliative care patients. The basis of this is as follows.

- Every individual is unique.
- In order to be treated properly, symptoms and illness must be understood in the context of the emotional, social and spiritual circumstances of that individual.
- Life has meaning and the events in it have a purpose.
- Illness can provide an opportunity for change.

It is sometimes thought that a patient or problem can be treated with either conventional/orthodox therapies, or complementary therapies, but not both. Simiarly, it is sometimes supposed that a practitioner of, say, acupuncture, will have entirely abandoned conventional concepts of physiology and of the causes of illness and health. In fact, neither of these suppositions is correct. Complementary therapies often work very well when added to conventional treatments, as their name implies.

Use in palliative care

- The strategies employed by many complementary therapies ensure a continued positive approach to the situation. It is never the case that 'We can't do anything more for you'.
- In many therapies there is an emphasis on physical contact. Attention is therefore drawn to touch and interaction. This is in contrast with the fear or awkwardness of contact between carers and patient that sometimes exist, usually unintentionally. This emphasis on physical touch tends to be absent in a more intensive conventional medical setting. Therapies can sometimes be taught to carers, thereby increasing their involvement with the patient.

- Most of these therapies are less dependent on technology and give more attention to the environment around the patient, appreciating its importance in the situation and using or altering the sight, smell, sound and feel of these surroundings to the patient's benefit.
- Therapists usually appreciate that a diagnosis is not as important as the effect that it has on the patient in terms of their own assessment of loss of function and of quality of life.
- The approach is more patient centred than, say, that traditionally taken by conventional hospital medicine. Complementary therapies are usually more holistic and help to acknowledge the patient's full human identity and autonomy. This is just the time in life when someone is likely to feel loss of autonomy and identity due to the physical changes and altered self-image that occur.

These ideas are very largely in keeping with the philosophy of palliative care itself.

Potential concerns and difficulties

Complementary therapies can raise some problems with regard to their use.

Personal responsibility for health problems

The principle that behaviour, surroundings and actions can be used to affect health status can backfire if a patient ends up thinking that it is partly their own fault that they are ill, due to failure to try harder in some way. For example, a patient with advanced cancer who is suffering from anorexia may feel that they *ought* to be eating more. Complementary therapy practitioners need to be aware of this pitfall.

Conventional assessment must go on

Complementary treatment could potentially make it more difficult to recognise the developing symptoms of a treatable complication (e.g. hypercalcaemia). Continued vigilance by the usual conventional practitioners is still necessary.

Belief conflicts

There may be conflicting health models in the minds of those on the professional side of the patient's care. In addition, conventional health workers may mean something slightly different to a complementary therapist when using a particular word or phrase. Care is needed to ensure high-quality communication between carers. Once some familiarity and understanding has developed between the various parties, a growing degree of trust will be present which helps to eliminate this problem.

A similar problem can occur among the patient's relatives and carers if their beliefs about complementary therapies differ. This can potentially lead to fragmentation of care and communication problems between carers, and the patient could end up in a stressful 'piggy-in-the-middle' situation.

Organisation and supervision

Many complementary therapists will not be working within the conventional structure of the NHS. In palliative care, volunteer workers are common and some complementary therapists may fall into this category. For each patient, there needs to be someone responsible for the effective 'employment' of the complementary therapist. This person should be able to set out lines of clinical responsibility and to reach agreement with the therapist about their qualifications, job description and the limits of their practice. Some nurses in hospices are also trained in complementary therapies, which makes such arrangements simpler. Most therapies now have recognised governing bodies that can offer advice on some of these issues.

Acupuncture

Acupuncture as practised by most Western doctors involves the placing of fine needles in meridians (energy channels) situated in different parts of the skin to produce effects distant from the point of insertion. There is a steadily growing base of increasingly sound evidence for the efficacy of acupuncture in the treatment of various symptoms. However, much of this evidence has not been collected from palliative care patients.

Acupuncture works by stimulation of nerve fibres. Numerous substances are released local to each needle. Some of these are analgesic, but many of them have other properties. There is a very low incidence of side-effects in acupuncture.

Table 6.1 lists some of the substances released and their effects.[1]

Table 6.1   Substances released by acupuncture and their effects

Opioids Endorphins	Pain relief
Serotonin	Pain relief, lifting of mood
Oxytocin	Pain relief, sedation
Adrenocorticotropic hormone	Anti-inflammatory
Changes in opioid gene regulation (method unclear)	Possible cause of prolongation of treatment effects seen
Immune system effects (substance unknown)	Possible enhancement of immune function which could be beneficial in patients with cancer

Potential uses of acupuncture in palliative care

Pain

Acupuncture has been shown to be of benefit in both acute and chronic pain. It could be considered as a treatment option, especially if a patient fails to respond well to conventional drugs or is suffering from persistent side-effects of them. Acupuncture may allow a lower dose of drug to be effective and may improve pain control. The main problem at present is that effects are seldom prolonged, so treatment needs to be frequent and ongoing.

Breathlessness (dyspnoea)

Significant benefits have been shown in the treatment of breathlessness and the anxiety that accompanies it. If necessary, needles can be left *in situ* for up to 2 weeks at a time and stimulated by the patient when needed.

Anxiety

Acupuncture seems to be particularly effective in treating anxiety and stress, both of which are common in this group of patients.

Radio-necrotic ulcers

Ulcers associated with radiotherapy damage to the skin are very difficult to heal. Acupuncture may improve the likelihood of them healing.

Dry mouth

Dry mouth due to salivary gland damage, typically occurring after head or neck radiotherapy, is persistent and often quite severe. Acupuncture can improve salivary flow in this situation.

Nausea and vomiting

Acupuncture has been shown to be useful in helping to control these symptoms, including the sometimes severe nausea and vomiting associated with chemotherapy.

Others

There are reports of successful use of acupuncture to treat hiccup, radiotherapy-associated proctitis (inflammation of the rectum, which is likely to cause pain, discharge and bleeding), itching and depression. However, more research, especially in palliative care patients, is needed to confirm this.

Contraindications to acupuncture in palliative care

1   In an area of spinal instability, as acupuncture may cause muscles to relax from their potentially protective state of spasm and thus increase the risk of spinal cord damage.
2   In a limb where lymphoedema is present.
3   In a patient with a severe clotting disorder.
4   Electro-acupuncture is contraindicated in a patient with a pacemaker.

Side-effects

Side-effects are rare, but can include the following:

* fainting
* bruising
* sedation
* infection at needle site
* tissue damage (e.g. take great care when using needles on the chest wall of a cachectic patient – it may be thinner than you think)
* acupuncture is possibly less effective in very weak and severely cachectic patients. The procedure itself may also be too traumatising for such patients unless very few needles are used.

Aromatherapy

Aromatherapy is the use of essential oils extracted from plants to treat illness and symptoms. These extracts can be administered in a number of different ways;

* massage on to the skin in a carrier oil – this may include a component that facilitates skin absorption. This is the most common method of use
* vaporisation in the patient's room – this can be useful if massage is inappropriate
* inhalations in hot water
* in compresses that are applied to specific areas of pain or inflammation
* in baths.

Different essential oils are thought to be useful for different purposes. For example:

* lavender for insomnia
* peppermint for nausea
* sandalwood for its relaxant, calming, sedative properties
* eucalyptus – refreshing, stimulating, good for certain respiratory problems.

A recent audit of aromatherapy and massage in a hospice offering these as complementary therapies noted the following points.

The reasons for seeking help were, among others:

1   needing relaxation (71%)
2   being in pain (22%)
3   suffering anxiety (22%).

Reported benefits included the following:

1   relaxation (95%)
2   increased sense of well-being (85%)
3   interestingly – time to talk (73%)
4   coping better with symptoms (71%)
5   greater ease of joint movement (51%).

Contraindications

Some essential oils are potentially harmful to a developing embryo/fetus, particularly during the first 13 weeks of pregnancy. Potentially pregnant women must avoid them, which could create problems for some patients' carers.

Massage

Massage alone also has some reported benefits. It has been found to decrease anxiety levels in some patients.

It also appears to help to relieve pain in some patients. Specialist massage and bandaging are used for treatment of lymphoedema. Massage is claimed to help the following symptoms:

• insomnia
• fatigue
• agitation and restlessness.

It is particularly helpful in that it provides physical contact with the patient. Someone with advanced cancer may have few good experiences from day to day, so positive interaction with another person is likely to become much more important. This emphasises the fact that they are very much a person at a time when their self-image is poor, and so decreases their isolation.[2]

Visualisation and imagery

This is the use of mental imagery and imagination to create and focus on pictures in the mind (e.g. of a favourite beautiful place), to beneficially influence the patient's subjective experience of their symptoms and disease.

Together with relaxation techniques, visualisation and imagery can be taught on an individual basis to the patient, who can then put them into practice whenever necessary. It is suggested that they can produce benefits when dealing with pain, nausea and vomiting.

References

1 Filshie J (2000) Acupuncture in palliative care. *Eur J Palliative Care.* **7**: 41–4.
2 Autton N (1996) The use of touch in palliative care. *Eur J Palliative Care.* **3**: 121–4.

Sources of useful information

Aromatherapy Organisations Council, PO Box 19834, London SE25 6WF. Tel: 020 8251 7912. Fax: 020 8251 7942. Website: http://www.aoc.uk.net
British Massage Therapy Council, 17 Rymers Lane, Oxford OX4 3JU. Website: http://www.bmtc.co.uk

Further reading

- Autton N (1996) The use of touch in palliative care. *Eur J Palliative Care.* **3**: 121–4.
- Filshie J (2000) Acupuncture in palliative care. *Eur J Palliative Care.* **7**: 41–4.
- Pietroni P (2000/2001) Complementary medicine: an overview. In: *RCGP Members' Reference Book 2000/2001.* Royal College of General Practitioners, London.
- Vickers A (1998) *Massage and Aromatherapy: a guide for health professionals.* Stanley Thornes, Cheltenham.
- Vickers A and Zollman C (1999) ABC of complementary medicine. Massage therapies. *BMJ.* **319**: 1254–7.
- Vickers A and Zollman C (1999) ABC of complementary medicine. Unconventional approaches to nutritional medicine. *BMJ.* **319**: 1419–22.
- Vickers A and Zollman C (1999) ABC of complementary medicine. Complementary medicine and the doctor. *BMJ.* **319**: 1558–61.

Useful websites

Further advice on acupuncture and on finding an acupuncturist is available from the British Acupuncture Council, 63 Jeddo Road, London W12 9HQ. Tel: 020 8735 0400. Email: info@acupuncture.org.uk. Website: www.acupuncture.org.uk
More advice about acupuncture and finding a local practitioner is available from the British Medical Acupuncture Society. Website: www.medical-acupuncture.co.uk

Acknowledgements

I would like to thank Viv Brown DipAc, MTAS, an experienced acupuncturist in Leamington Spa, and SN Chris Emerson, who practises aromatherapy at Myton Hamlet Hospice in Warwick, for useful discussions.

CHAPTER 7

Out-of-hours and emergency palliative care

Dan Munday

Introduction

Palliative care for patients in the community should be available 24 hours a day, 365 days of the year. What happens during the 119 hours of the week which fall outside the working hours of 8a.m.–6p.m. Monday to Friday is attracting much debate. A number of papers have appeared in both general practice and palliative care journals highlighting the issue of out-of-hours palliative care, and it is discussed in the recent Department of Health out-of-hours report. In March 2001, Macmillan Cancer Relief published *Out-of-Hours Palliative Care in the Community*, the report of a working group drawn from primary care and specialist palliative care, whose remit was to examine the issues and to highlight good practice. This report highlights the main issues and gives examples of good practice.

In order to provide good palliative care, there is a need for a well co-ordinated service with good communication between all professionals involved in patient care. These services involve both members of the primary care team (principally general practitioners and district nurses) and doctors and nurses in specialist palliative care teams. The other vital features of good out-of-hours palliative care include nurses available to care for patients at home over a 24-hour period, and access to beds in palliative care units for patients who are no longer able to stay in their own homes.

Variation in care

There is evidence of great variation throughout the UK in the provision of both primary and specialist palliative care services out of hours. A recent survey of GP out-of-hours co-operative medical directors suggested that in only about half of the UK is there access to 24-hour district nursing services. In addition, 80% of respondents claimed to have difficulty in arranging 24-hour nursing services at short notice. Although the majority reported that specialist palliative care services were available in their locality, only about 50% knew of an out-of-hours specialist advice service. Finally, very few co-operatives are able to access specialist palliative care beds out of hours.

GP co-operatives

Since 1995, out-of-hours GP co-operatives have become the commonest way for general practitioners to provide out-of-hours care for their patients. Many comments both from specialist palliative care services and from those in primary care with a special interest in palliative care cast doubt on the ability of co-operatives to provide adequate care for palliative care patients. These comments have been largely based on personal opinion and anecdote, as little research has been conducted in this area. There is also no published evidence to support the notion that out-of-hours palliative care provided by GPs within practice rotas is superior to that provided by co-operatives.

This chapter will explore the issues surrounding the provision of good palliative care out of hours. It will suggest how primary care teams, particularly co-operatives and deputising services, can ensure high-quality care for all terminally ill patients, and it will highlight specific examples of good practice. Finally, there will be a discussion of clinical conditions which may present a particular problem to medical and nursing staff out of hours, and ways in which these problems may be best managed will be suggested.

Organisation of out-of-hours palliative care

At a series of workshops in 1999 and 2000, the National Association of GP Co-operatives (NAGPC) produced guidelines for their members on the provision of excellent palliative care. These were designed to highlight important areas of palliative care and to provide a framework for co-operatives to develop locally appropriate guidelines. The principles expressed are transferable to other models of care, particularly deputising services and extended practice rotas. Unless local guidelines are developed for dealing with calls coming from palliative care patients or their carers, these patients may not receive appropriate care.

Many areas now have GP palliative care facilitators, often funded and supported by Macmillan Cancer Relief. These practising GPs, who have a special interest and often a postgraduate qualification in palliative care, are a useful resource for developing guidelines, assisting with clinical governance activity and providing education. Many co-operatives have also accessed palliative care specialists to assist in these areas.

Guidelines should be developed locally by co-operatives, deputising services and other providers of out-of-hours care. Several important areas need to be considered by these guidelines.

Issues relating to 'out-of-hours' palliative care (based on NAGPC guidelines)

Communication

Patients prefer to receive personal continuity of care. Although it is impossible for a GP to provide 24-hour care personally, patients or their carers are reassured by the knowledge that a GP has personally passed over information. For example, an on-call GP is able to say 'Dr Smith has told us about your father's condition. What seems to be the problem tonight?'. A robust system is needed to ensure effective communication of patient information between the primary care team and the co-operative, deputising or other out-of-hours service, and between professionals within that service.

- *Information into the organisation.* Many co-operatives have introduced fax forms to facilitate a flow of important information from practices to the co-operative (*see* Box 7.1). Auditing the effect of the introduction of one such form showed an improvement in communication.
- *Information within the organisation.* Should a follow-up call be made regarding a patient, the professional responding to this second call must have full information regarding the first call. Patients and their carers are not reassured if two doctors from the same service do not seem to have communicated!
- *Information from the organisation to the practice.* It is essential that information regarding contact with all palliative care patients out of hours reaches their primary care team swiftly to ensure continuity of care. Many co-operatives fax* the consultation record for all contacts to the practice by the beginning of the next working day.

NHS Direct

Part of the health development strategy of the present government has been the introduction of NHS Direct. A caller to NHS Direct will first of all speak to a specially trained nurse who will triage the call. Advice is given for self-care or the most appropriate course of action with regard to seeking further help (e.g. calling the out-of-hours GP, calling for an ambulance or visiting the GP the following day). The nurse follows set protocols presented to him or her in a computer-assisted decision support system.

There has been some concern about the appropriateness of the advice given to palliative care patients as a result of this system. There is also a danger that patients and their carers will feel that their care is being passed from 'pillar to post' and becoming increasingly anonymised. Many co-operatives are now using NHS Direct as their triage system, calls being made directly to the co-operative as appropriate. If NHS Direct is the normal 'front end' for out-of-hours contacts for patients, it is imperative that information about palliative care patients is passed on to NHS Direct by practices.

Protocols for care

Once the call regarding a terminally ill patient has been received, it needs to be dealt with appropriately by all personnel, from the receptionist who receives the call to the healthcare professionals involved in dealing with the patient right up to

---

*Fax is likely to be superseded by electronic mail through the NHSnet.

Box 7.1 Example of a fax form for information to send to a GP co-operative

FAX number

TO CO-OPERATIVE PATIENT FILE

Terminally ill patient   Date:

Name/age:	
Address: GP and practice:	
Diagnosis primary, secondary spread and complicating conditions: Present (*and proposed future*) treatment:	
Bed available:	
Main carer and relationship (contact phone number):	
Other comments:	

the time when information is passed back to the patient's practice. A multidisciplinary group may be the most effective forum for developing protocols covering all aspects of palliative care delivery by the organisation, with representatives from all professionals who will be involved in their implementation. The following issues should be addressed.

- *Who takes the call?* Is it passed on to the GP, the district nurse or the specialist nurse? Does the responsible professional know that they are to take such calls? Do they know how calls should be triaged?
- *Do all such patients receive a visit?* Anecdotal reports do exist that illustrate how patients have been inappropriately asked to attend 'on-call centres' when they were clearly housebound and extremely unwell.
- *What should be the response time for such calls?* Although response should always be based on clinical need, patients and their carers are often anxious and need reassurance. Having to wait two or three hours before a visit is made merely heightens this anxiety and may lead to unnecessary admission.
- *Which drugs and what equipment are carried by doctors?* This area can be addressed with the help of professionals with a special interest in palliative care. The introduction of such a list could represent an opportunity to provide teaching on symptom control. There are many examples of good practice in this area.
- *If a syringe driver is needed, who will provide this? Does the service have access to syringe drivers when they are needed?* In the majority of areas, district nurses are responsible for the management of syringe drivers. If nurses are not available on a 24-hour basis, who is then responsible for the service? Lack of such a service leads to a failure of appropriate care and is an important cause of potentially avoidable admission.
- *Is a dedicated palliative care team an option?* Larger co-operatives might decide to form 'rapid-response palliative care teams' with special expertise and access to specialist equipment and drugs. The team may consist entirely of primary care professionals with a special interest in palliative care, or it may include members of specialist palliative care teams.
- *If a patient requires specialist input, is this available?* The providers of specialist palliative care should be asked to provide clear instructions on how to access their services out of hours. This information needs to be disseminated to all professionals who might potentially need to access a specialist service. Since it might be uncommon for individual practitioners to require specialist advice, regular reminders of its availability should back up the written protocol.

Access to controlled drugs

It is unfortunate that recent high-profile cases within the UK involving the misuse of strong opioid drugs have led to great public and professional anxiety regarding the use of controlled drugs. Although the use of these drugs needs to be well regulated, tight restrictions on their storage and transport may lead to problems in ensuring their availability for palliative care patients. Out-of-hours services need to ensure that patients are provided with appropriate drugs swiftly and safely.

Solutions include the following.

- Co-operatives store controlled drugs in the on-call centre with a local pharmacy updating stock on a regular basis. The regulations for the storage of controlled drugs are complex, and they differ between Scotland and England. A Home Office Licence may be necessary in England.
- An on-call rota of chemists who stock all potentially necessary drugs is locally available.
- Hospital or hospice pharmacies provide drugs as needed by arrangement with the out-of-hours service.

The law relating to the prescription and supply of controlled drugs is complex. Before a system for the supply of drugs becomes operational, its legalities need to be checked by the co-operative management team in order to avoid unlawful practices.

Audit and education

Critics of present out-of-hours arrangements for primary care in the UK cite the palliative care patient as being disadvantaged. However, out-of-hours co-operatives do present a real opportunity for pursuing standardised excellent care, rather than highly variable care depending on the knowledge, skills and attitudes of individual practitioners. In my experience, the co-operative as a forum for sharing ideas and examples of good practice by members is one of the great opportunities of the present system. More formally, however, all out-of-hours services do need to invest time and effort not only in protocol development but also in audit to ensure high-quality care.

Arranging educational events on all aspects of emergency medical care can be highly successful. These events should address palliative care issues, including symptom control and the recognition and management of treatable disease complications. Since many GPs have not received formal training in palliative care, such educational events will be valuable for 'in-hours' practice, too.

An example of a co-operative which has invested in the development of out-of-hours palliative care and its governance is shown in Box 7.2.

Emergency palliative care

One of the cardinal rules of good palliative care is to try to anticipate problems which may occur. Ensuring that patients have adequate supplies of medication is paramount, and warning patients and their carers of possible complications and what to do 'in an emergency' is good practice. Primary care teams should make sure that clear instructions are left, preferably in writing, and that a full hand-over has been made to the on-call service (as above). Unfortunately, back-up services are not always available out of hours, and on-call primary care teams are left to cope with problems with which they may be unfamiliar. Even in the absence of a formal out-of-hours advice service, most hospice inpatient units are very willing to give advice, as are oncology ward nurses.

Box 7.2   Example of good practice in the area of palliative care in a co-operative – Grampian Doctors-On-Call Service (GDOCS)

April 1996 – GDOCS established. Palliative care drugs box developed by local GP palliative care facilitator. Boxes available in each on-call vehicle and at the emergency centre.

November 1997 – Multidisciplinary audit of communication between GPs and co-operative regarding known terminally ill patients. District nurses involved in identifying terminally ill patients. Results showed that the co-operative had received notification regarding only 20% of terminally ill patients from GPs.

January 1998 – Fax form introduced after a meeting of co-operative members, with unanimous agreement to use the form. Regular mailings to member practices used to highlight need to use forms for such patients.

September 1998 – Audit repeated. For 55% of terminally ill patients a fax form had now been received from GPs. Regular reminders continue to be a feature of mailings to practices.

September to November 1999 – Audit of symptom control decisions comparing decision with best practice (from local guidelines); 75% of decisions relating to pain were judged to be appropriate. Fewer decisions regarding control of other symptoms (e.g. nausea and vomiting) were judged to be appropriate. Overall, 65% of decisions were judged to be appropriate, with only 15% being judged to be contrary to guidelines. A different choice of drug or route of administration could have improved the remainder (20% of decisions).

February 2000 – Half-day training in symptom control in palliative care arranged by co-operative and GP palliative care facilitator, with facilitator and local palliative care consultant running an interactive teaching session. This session formed part of a programme of training in other aspects of out-of-hours primary care.

Patient care may suffer due to ineffective teamworking. Many district nurses have considerable experience in palliative care and have a sound knowledge base with regard to symptom control, including the use of opioid drugs and anti-emetics. Unfortunately, it is not unusual to hear experienced district nurses express frustration at the attitude of some medical colleagues out of hours, who seem to be reluctant to visit a patient or to receive advice from the district nurse. Discussion of management issues with other members of the team in an open and non-judgemental way is central to effective and safe palliative care. However, teamworking is based on mutual respect for the professionalism of others and the ability to accept that they may have skills and experience which we do not possess.

Not all situations can be foreseen, and often problems occur without warning. We shall now consider some of the more common emergency situations which may arise or come to light out of hours.

Severe pain

This is perhaps the commonest 'emergency' in the palliative care setting. Whilst it is always important to plan ahead and to make sure that patients have sufficient supplies of analgesics and other drugs for weekends and bank holidays, unforeseen problems with pain control are not uncommon.

- *The pain may worsen.* Patients should have adequate supplies of 'breakthrough' medication, even if this has not been previously required. Patients and their carers should be given clear instructions on how to administer this medication.
- *A 'new' pain may emerge.* This may be due to a variety of causes, including pathological fracture, bleeding into or torsion of a tumour, erosion into a nerve, etc. The nature of the pain should be elucidated and the appropriate management decisions made.
- *The route of administration may no longer be effective.* Patients who are taking oral medication may start to vomit or have difficulty in swallowing. Those who are using transdermal patches may become 'sweaty', so that the patch falls off. In such cases the availability of a syringe driver, the skills necessary to use it and the staff to monitor it are of vital importance.

Vomiting

It is not uncommon for patients with vomiting to be admitted to acute hospital beds only to have their vomiting immediately controlled by the judicious use of anti-emetics in a syringe driver. These admissions may be regarded as 'unnecessary' and can be distressing for patients and relatives alike. Anticipation of nausea and vomiting following the introduction of opioid analgesics or an increase in their dosage constitutes good palliative care. It is appropriate to prescribe anti-emetics in this situation, giving clear instructions to start the drug and to take it regularly as soon as the patient feels any nausea. Such action may help to avoid the need for parenteral drugs.

Hypercalcaemia

Around 10–20% of patients with malignant disease develop hypercalcaemia. The commonest cancers in which hypercalcaemia may occur are squamous-cell lung cancer, breast cancer, genito-urinary cancer, lymphoma and myeloma. It may also occur in squamous-cell head and neck cancers and malignant melanoma, but is said to be less common in prostate, stomach and colon cancers.

Hypercalcaemia is easily missed, since it may develop quite suddenly and its symptoms can be mistaken for general deterioration. With mild hypercalcaemia, the patient may appear lethargic and may complain of anorexia, nausea and constipation and appear generally withdrawn. As the serum calcium level rises, the patient will become more drowsy and delirious, and may show signs of paralytic ileus. Eventually, unconsciousness and cardiovascular collapse will ensue. Signs of severe hypercalcaemia may be the first presentation, and the condition needs to be treated as an emergency, otherwise the patient's condition may deteriorate rapidly, with death occurring due to cardiac arrhythmias. Hypercalcaemia should always be suspected if a patient has *refractory* nausea, constipation and pain. The classical symptoms of polyuria and polydipsia seem to occur relatively infrequently.

Treating hypercalcaemia

Deciding whether to treat hypercalcaemia actively may be difficult. Patients who have been otherwise reasonably well until the onset of hypercalcaemia should be offered full treatment, since it will help to control refractory symptoms and also possibly lengthen the patient's life. In a patient who has been progressively deteriorating, treatment may not be so appropriate. However, it must be considered whether this deterioration has in fact been a result of the undiagnosed hypercalcaemia from the outset. Patients who have been previously treated are likely to become hypercalcaemic again. Unfortunately, treatment is often less successful with each successive attempt. Treatment options should always be discussed with the patient and their relatives before a decision is made. If a patient has been previously hypercalaemic and has received treatment, it is preferable to discuss with them their feelings about further treatment in the event of a subsequent episode, rather than leave the decision until the problem has recurred.

Treatment will normally require admission, although some specialist community teams are now treating such patients in their homes. Hypercalcaemic patients are dehydrated, and initial treatment must always involve rehydration. Following this, the administration of intravenous bisphosphonates is often successful in bringing the calcium levels under control. If the symptoms are mild, taking a blood sample for calcium, albumin and electrolytes in the patient's home and deciding on admission once the results are available is probably the most reasonable course of action. It is preferable that treatment should start within 24 hours, but there is no greater urgency unless the serum calcium level is above 3 mmol/L. If the patient appears to have the symptoms of severe hypercalcaemia or the serum calcium level is above 3 mmol/L, it is advisable to admit them and start treatment immediately.

Severe shortness of breath

Shortness of breath is a common problem in advanced cancer, and studies suggest that 50–70% of patients suffer from it. The causes are varied and include the following:

- destruction of lung tissue by lung cancer or secondary spread
- obstruction of bronchus by tumour (intrinsic or extrinsic) or secretions
- upper airway obstruction by (inoperable) head and neck tumour

- pleural effusion
- mesothelioma
- pneumonia
- anaemia
- heart failure
- pulmonary embolism
- superior vena caval obstruction (SVCO)
- lymphangitis carcinomatosa.

Patients with non-malignant diagnoses who require palliative care often suffer from breathlessness as well. Common non-malignant diseases that lead to breathlessness include the following:

- end-stage cardiac failure
- end-stage obstructive airways disease
- fibrosing alveolitis
- motor neurone disease
- multiple sclerosis
- AIDS.

Breathlessness can be particularly distressing and difficult to treat. The situation may deteriorate rapidly, with the patient becoming anxious, resulting in a vicious cycle of breathlessness, panic and worsening breathlessness.

Management
This must be holistic in its approach, with not only physical and psychological aspects but also social implications and spiritual effects being addressed. Although a thorough assessment must be made in the search for a treatable cause, such as pleural effusion or anaemia, in the emergency situation the treatment is common to all causes of breathlessness. Treatment of specific causes is beyond the scope of this chapter.

Physical management
- *Oxygen therapy*. This is not always successful, and there is little evidence that the benefit in lung cancer patients corresponds to the degree of hypoxia. A stream of air (e.g. from a fan or sitting by an open window) may palliate some patients to the same extent.
- *Opioid analgesics*. These are a mainstay of treatment, taking advantage of their respiratory depressant effect. A small dose of oral morphine (e.g. 2.5–5 mg 4-hourly) may be sufficient, especially in opioid-naive patients. Diamorphine given parenterally is three times more potent than oral morphine, so doses as small as 1.25 mg may be effective in this situation. For persistent severe breathlessness, continuous subcutaneous infusion of diamorphine 5–10 mg over 24 hours is often beneficial. There is no advantage in using nebulised morphine, which may induce bronchospasm.

- *Benzodiazepines*. These can be useful for treating anxiety, especially in an attempt to break the cycle of panic and breathlessness. When given in small doses they do not suppress respiration, and they can be safely given to the severely breathless patient. Lorazepam (1–2 mg) may be given orally or sublingually. It has a rapid onset, its effects last for about 2 or 3 hours and it can be especially helpful for acute panic attacks. Midazolam (2.5–5 mg) is given parenterally and is useful for patients who are unable to swallow. Diazepam is longer acting and useful for patients who are suffering repeated panic attacks or sustained anxiety associated with breathlessness. It is effective in doses of 2–5 mg 8-hourly.
- *Nebuliser with bronchodilators or normal saline*. This may help in bronchospasm and in weakened patients, where it can aid the expectoration of viscid sputum.

All drugs which cause sedation are potentially dangerous to patients with *upper airways obstruction*. They should be avoided if there is scope for overcoming the obstruction (e.g. with a tracheostomy). Clearly, for patients who are at the terminal stage and in whom no further corrective treatment is possible, judicious use of opioids and benzodiazepines may be made, but small increments should be given in an attempt to avoid total upper airway obstruction. Fortunately, this situation is rare and treatment should not be withheld for this reason. This is clearly one area in which specialist help may be of benefit, and the 'doctrine of double effect' allows the physician to administer adequate palliative treatment.

Psychological management
- The patient should be reassured. The anxiety associated with severe shortness of breath should be tackled by the confident and reassuring manner of the attending healthcare professionals. Fears and concerns should be addressed openly and honestly, and a clear explanation of the link between panic and breathlessness can help the patient to understand what is happening. The patient may be reminded about breathing exercises.
- The relatives should be reassured, given a full explanation and their help enlisted in providing a safe, reassuring environment for the patient.
- Moving a patient to a hospice unit may help by providing him or her with a safe environment while investigation of the breathlessness and optimisation of the symptom control are undertaken.

Social management
Adapting the patient's home to allow them to function within their restricted abilities should be addressed in the long term.

Spiritual management
Patients with persistent breathlessness often become very disillusioned and questioning. Requests for euthanasia in this situation are not uncommon. Spiritual support is of extreme importance, and should be given to suit the patient's needs and beliefs.

Superior vena caval obstruction (SVCO)

Pressure on the thin-walled superior vena cava from tumour in the mediastinum, most commonly lung, but also lymphoma, breast and other solid tumours, may lead to obstruction of blood flow from the head and neck back to the heart. Occasionally it is accompanied by intravascular tumour. The onset is often acute, patients presenting with acute symptoms of shortness of breath, headache, swelling of soft tissues in the head, neck and arms, dilated veins and petechial haemorrhages in severe cases. It is not uncommon for SVCO to be the presenting syndrome in patients with lung cancer, so it should be considered in any at-risk patient who presents with these symptoms. Urgent admission should be arranged for confirmation and management of the condition.

Chest X-ray will show a widened mediastinum, often with other features of lung cancer. CT scanning will demonstrate a compressed superior vena cava, and occasionally the presence of clot or tumour within it. For patients in whom SVCO is the presenting complaint, bronchoscopy may be performed to secure a tissue diagnosis.

Management

As in all situations of impaired breathing, patients will prefer to sit upright. Treatment consists of high-dose steroids (e.g. dexamethasone 16 mg daily) and radiotherapy. Recently, stenting of the SVC has become more common, and often gives good and rapid results.

Spinal cord compression (SCC)

This is relatively common, occurring in 3–5% of patients with advanced cancer, although the individual GP will see only one case every 5–10 years. However, a high index of suspicion is needed, since early diagnosis is paramount for achieving a good outcome.

SCC may be due to metastases in a vertebral body expanding to fill the epidural space and impinging on the spinal cord. This is often accompanied by vertebral body collapse. Other causes include tumour growing through inter-vertebral foramina, and metastases developing within the epidural space itself. Around 40% of cases of SCC occur in prostate, breast and lung cancer. Other common causes are myeloma, renal and thyroid carcinoma, melanoma and lymphoma. Any vertebral level might be affected. The commonest site is in the thoracic vertebrae, followed by the lumbar and finally cervical vertebrae. Multiple levels occur in 20% of cases.

Presentation may be insidious, with the patient being 'off their legs'. SCC should be considered in any patient who has back pain radiating into the limbs, limb weakness, paraesthesia, sensory disturbance or urinary sphincter dysfunction. Pain is the commonest symptom, with 90% of patients reporting pain when questioned retrospectively after diagnosis. Patients with compression below the lower end of the spinal cord suffer from the separate but related 'cauda equina syndrome'. Patients with sacral level compression may only show signs of sensory disturbance in the perineal region.

Diagnosis of SCC is confirmed by MRI scan. Admission should not be delayed if the diagnosis is suspected, and it is preferable to speak directly to the palliative medicine physician or oncologist on call, since the urgency of the situation is sadly not always recognised on general medical or surgical wards. Treatment is with high-dose steroids initially, followed by radiotherapy. Some specialist centres are achieving very impressive results with emerging spinal surgery techniques. If there is a high index of suspicion, and in the rare event of admission being delayed, 16 mg dexamethasone should be commenced in the community.

Once neurological signs are established, the likelihood of a good functional outcome following treatment is drastically reduced. Unfortunately, symptoms are often discovered to have been present for several weeks before diagnosis.

Pathological fracture

This should be suspected if there is severe pain in a long bone, often of sudden onset and worsened by movement. For patients who are sufficiently fit, treatment is by stabilisation of the fracture with operative fixation followed by radiotherapy. Patients who are unfit for surgery may require admission to a palliative care unit because of the difficulty of nursing a patient with an unstable fracture.

It is often possible to diagnose impending pathological fracture by recognising worsening pain, particularly on movement, presumably due to small cortical fractures through the site of the metastasis. Many orthopaedic surgeons will stabilise these fractures prophylactically to prevent the inevitable full fracture from occurring. Patients in the community who are found to have symptoms suggestive of impending fracture should be admitted for assessment.

Treatment of pain due to pathological fractures is with strong opioids and NSAIDs. Additional pain on movement (e.g. for personal care and nursing procedures) is extremely common and requires short-acting analgesia. The recently introduced transmucosal fentanyl is an opioid with rapid onset and short duration of action, and it is proving extremely useful in this situation. Nerve blocks, such as femoral nerve and brachial plexus, may be useful for achieving analgesia for transporting the patient, but these require skills which may not be readily available in the community.

Terminal agitation

Up to 75% of patients with terminal cancer develop mental clouding and delirium during the last few days of life. The patient and their relatives may become severely distressed in this situation. A cause for the delirium should be sought, although often no obvious cause can be found. Urinary retention, lying in a wet bed following incontinence, and uncontrolled pain are all common problems which may be implicated, and these should be excluded and managed appropriately. Hypercalcaemia, electrolyte imbalance, urinary or chest infection, hypoxia and drug side-effects, particularly those due to steroids and opioids, are also common causes. The extent to which these problems should be investigated and treated depends on the previous condition of the patient. Assessment should be thorough, involving discussions with the family or other informal carers and community nurses who are looking after the patient.

Management should be within a safe, protective environment, avoiding over-stimulation, and with the reassuring presence of familiar relatives or friends who have themselves been briefed and reassured about what is happening to the patient. Haloperidol 5–20 mg daily in divided doses may help to improve mental clouding, while lorazepam 0.5–1 mg will help to sedate a distressed patient. Patients who are unable to take oral medication may be treated with midazolam 5–60 mg over a period of 24 hours in a syringe driver. Since it is difficult to predict the correct dose of sedative, the drug should be started at the lower end of the scale and titrated upwards according to response.

A specialist team should assess patients in whom control of agitation proves difficult, and admission is often necessary, especially if the carers are distressed and unable to cope further.

Massive haemorrhage

Fortunately this is quite rare, but it is an extremely distressing terminal event. Causes include haemoptysis, haematemesis and the erosion of major superficial blood vessels, especially the carotid arteries in fungating head and neck tumours. Minor bleeding may occur as a 'warning' of a more major bleed to come, and can often be controlled by local pressure over the bleeding point, swabs soaked in 1:100 000 adrenaline solution and the use of tranexamic acid. Catastrophic bleeding should be masked by using dark towels and by sedating the patient with diamorphine 5–10 mg and midazolam 5–10 mg.

Massive haemorrhage is an extremely distressing event for the patient, their relatives and the clinical staff. It is often better to admit patients who are at risk of such bleeding to specialist units where appropriate management may be started immediately should haemorrhage occur. If the patient and their carers want the patient to remain at home, the problems should be broached sensitively and carefully to forewarn everyone concerned but to avoid unnecessary anxiety. The equipment and drugs necessary for the treatment of haemorrhage should be kept in the home, and if possible 24-hour nursing care should be arranged. Carers should be given clear instructions about who to call in the event of an emergency, and out-of-hours services must be briefed.

Conclusions

Out of hours can be a difficult time for patients and their carers. Although it is impossible for healthcare professionals to provide personal continuity of care, well-organised multidisciplinary out-of-hours services with access to important information that provide care in a sensitive and efficient manner can compensate for lack of personal continuity. Healthcare practitioners should be particularly aware of emergency conditions which may occur unexpectedly in terminally ill patients, and they should be able to manage these conditions swiftly and appropriately. Prompt action can alleviate much suffering, and may even prevent a premature death.

Further reading

- Barclay S, Rogers M and Todd C (1997) Communication between GPs and co-operatives is poor for terminally ill patients. *BMJ.* **315**: 1235–6.
- Department of Health (2000) *Raising Standards for Patients: new partnerships in out-of-hours care (independent review).* Department of Health, London.
- Doyle D, Hanks GW and MacDonald N (eds) (1998) *The Oxford Textbook of Palliative Medicine* (2e). Oxford University Press, Oxford.
- Kramer J (1992) Spinal cord compression in malignancy. *Palliative Med.* **6**: 202–11.
- Munday D, Carroll D and Douglas A (1999) GP out-of-hours co-operatives and the delivery of palliative care. *Br J Gen Pract.* **49**: 489.
- Shipman C and Dale J (1999) Responding to patients with particular needs. In: C Salisbury, J Dale and L Hallam (eds) *24-Hour Primary Care.* Radcliffe Medical Press, Oxford.
- Shipman C, Addington-Hall J, Barclay S *et al.* (2000) Providing palliative care in primary care: how satisfied are GPs and district nurses with current out-of-hours arrangements? *Br J Gen Pract.* **50**: 477–8.
- St Oswalds Hospice and Centre for Health Service Research (1995) *Palliative Care Crisis Response: needs assessment.* St Oswalds Hospice and Centre for Health Service Research, Newcastle upon Tyne.
- Thomas K (2000). Out-of-hours palliative care – bridging the gap. *Eur J Palliative Care.* **7**: 22–5.
- Thomas K (2001) *Out-of-Hours Palliative Care in the Community.* Macmillan Cancer Relief, London.

Useful website

National Association of GP Co-operatives; www.nagpc.org.uk

CHAPTER 8

Palliative care of non-malignant conditions
John Wilmot

Introduction

Most people die of conditions other than cancer. Can they gain anything from the philosophy or techniques of palliative care, as dealt with elsewhere in this book? Health professionals, influenced by the hospice movement, have developed and improved their skills in the care of patients with advanced cancer. Those suffering from malignant disease have had unpleasant symptoms relieved, have gained weeks or months of rewarding life, and have died peacefully. In principle, the lessons of palliative care should be highly applicable to a wide variety of conditions.

The clinical background

Various progressive diseases both shorten life and cause unpleasant symptoms. The differing challenges will be outlined first, and then appropriate responses to them will be considered.

Transition from active to palliative therapy

The question of when to cease active therapy (i.e. therapy aimed at achieving a cure) and initiate palliative care is a challenging one. This is less likely to be an issue for a GP than for a specialist, who is the practitioner more likely to be involved with the patient in this decision-making process.

It is difficult to define the point at which active therapy is unlikely to be of further benefit. It takes great skill to apply criteria which might indicate that a patient is incurable, and then to communicate and negotiate a decision involving informed consent with a patient to change from active to palliative treatment. It is a time of uncertainty for the patient, their relatives and healthcare professionals. The difficulty in defining this stage is thought to be one possible reason why many referrals to hospices occur late in the course of an incurable illness.

Given that most patients in Western cultures wish to know the truth, communication of a management plan based on informed consent and avoiding giving rise to false hope should be used to facilitate a smooth transition from active to adequate palliative therapy. However, with the explosion of investigative and therapeutic technologies, their appropriateness is often difficult to judge and negotiate, particularly if a potential for 'cure' remains. When treatment decisions are made, the balance of benefits must be weighed against the burdens and risks. Management negotiated with the patient should include treatment that achieves an acceptable balance between quality and quantity of life and what is best for the patient.

The boundaries between the two phases of care (active and palliative) are blurred, and a model of care based on respect for patient autonomy should ensure that the timing of the switch from curative to palliative care is appropriate. Defining the stage during an illness at which a patient is no longer curable is important if we are to try to avoid active therapy which is futile and to institute palliative therapy to alleviate symptoms and improve the quality of life that remains.

Heart failure

During the next decade, increasing numbers of people will both live and die with heart failure. This is partly a reflection of an ageing population, and partly an ironic result of widespread success in the prevention and treatment of acute cardiac disease. Most industrialised countries have experienced a decline in morbidity and mortality from ischaemic heart disease. However, larger numbers of people will survive acute cardiac episodes to live to older ages with a damaged heart (myocardium). Heart failure is much more common in old age, with nearly 20% of all those over 75 years of age being affected. Despite advances in the treatment of heart failure, the prognosis remains poor. Even among mildly affected patients, 5–10% will die each year, a figure that rises to 30–40% for patients with advanced disease.[1]

Research among individuals dying from heart failure has shown a wide range of symptoms, which are often distressing and last more than six months. These include poorly controlled dyspnoea, pain, nausea, constipation and low mood. At least one in six of these patients had symptoms as severe as those in patients with cancer being treated in hospices. Many of them seemed to know that they were dying, but open communication with health professionals was rare.[2]

Qualitative research among affected patients suggests that there is limited public understanding of heart failure. Patients who were interviewed appeared to need information about prognosis and their likely manner of death. Obstacles to communication with doctors included cognitive impairment and difficulties in getting to hospital to keep appointments. More disappointingly, some doctors seemed to believe that patients should not be told too much.[3]

Peripheral vascular disease is a common progressive disease. For severely affected individuals, surgery is the treatment of choice, but some of these patients decline intervention, are too frail, or may have a poor outcome after operation.

Chronic obstructive pulmonary disease (COPD)

Research indicates that those patients with end-stage COPD have a significantly impaired quality of life, perhaps worse than that of many patients with lung cancer. They generally lack the practical and emotional support that a diagnosis of malignant disease can attract from palliative care services.[4]

Degenerative neurological conditions

It is important to remember that dementia is the commonest degenerative neurological disease, whether it is of Alzheimer type or caused by a multi-infarction process. Anticholinergic drugs such as donepezil will become increasingly important, but their main effect is to postpone the time when long-term residential care will be needed.[5] Parkinson's disease is another important progressive disorder, with broadly similar care needs in its late stages. Multiple sclerosis eventually causes severe disability, as does motor neurone disease (MND, known in some countries as amyotrophic lateral sclerosis or ALS). The principles of palliative care have had a considerable impact in specialist neurological units, especially with the last of these disorders. In addition, hospices look after some patients with motor neurone disease and other advanced neurological illnesses, either for respite care or during the last few days of life.

Locomotor disorders

Joint disorders such as osteoarthritis or rheumatoid arthritis do not themselves shorten life, but they commonly contribute to pain and disability in older patients who have conditions such as heart failure or lung disease. Similar considerations apply to osteoporosis, which can cause very painful and disabling vertebral collapse fractures. Fractures of the femoral neck are a common consequence of osteoporosis, and they often result in a need for long-term residential care.

Infections

AIDS was first described in the USA in 1981, but the causative virus, human immunodeficiency virus (HIV), was only discovered in 1983.[6] By the end of 1999 there were 34.3 million people in the world living with HIV or AIDS. At present around 95% of all of these infections occur in developing countries and continents, particularly in sub-Saharan Africa.[6,7]

The use of combination antiretroviral therapy has resulted in an increased life expectancy among HIV sufferers.[6–8] This has increased the clinical dilemma of when to cease curative treatment and investigations and start palliative care.

The progression from HIV to AIDS can be determined using the WHO case definition for AIDS surveillance. A person over 12 years of age is considered to have AIDS if he or she has a positive HIV antibody test result together with one or more of the following conditions:

1   >10% body weight loss or cachexia, with diarrhoea, fever, or both, intermittent or constant, for at least a month, not known to be due to a condition unrelated to HIV infection

2 cryptococcal meningitis
3 pulmonary or extrapulmonary tuberculosis
4 Kaposi's sarcoma
5 neurological impairment that is sufficient to prevent independent daily activities and is not known to be due to a condition unrelated to HIV infection
6 candidiasis of the oesophagus
7 clinically diagnosed life-threatening or recurrent episodes of pneumonia, with or without aetiological confirmation
8 invasive cervical cancer.

However, there are a number of common conditions associated with AIDS which require active management until death. These are listed in Table 8.1.

Table 8.1 Management of problems associated with AIDS

Problem	Condition	Treatment
Oral	Oral candidiasis	Fluconazole or itraconazole
Lung	Kaposi's sarcoma	Symptomatic control – anxiolytics, opioids, oxygen
	Pneumocystis carinii pneumonia	Co-trimoxazole, pentamidine or dapsone
Ophthalmic	Conjunctivitis Cytomegalovirus retinitis	IV ganciclovir, foscarnet (must be prescribed by hospital doctor)
Nervous system	AIDS dementia complex	Combination therapy including zidovudine
Tumour related	Kaposi's sarcoma	Chemotherapy, radiotherapy
Gastrointestinal	Diarrhoea	Loperamide, hyosine butylbromide or ispaghula husk
	Constipation	Laxatives

vCJD

During the next decade, new variant Creutzfeld–Jacob disease (nvCJD), now referred to as variant Creutzfeld-Jacob disease (vCJD), will be an increasingly common cause of neurological deterioration and premature death, especially in the UK. Most affected individuals are currently cared for in hospital, but as their numbers increase, some may be found in nursing homes. The families and carers of these patients observe the rapid decline in the patient's mental state, which will cause a great deal of distress. Therefore the role of the primary healthcare team is to provide support for the patient and their carers. This can involve either providing access to honest and appropriate information on treatment and prognosis, or the provision of long-term palliative care.[9]

Dealing with symptoms

Pain

Simple analgesics used regularly remain an appropriate treatment for pain, even in advanced illness. The World Health Organization analgesic ladder suggests combination analgesia (paracetamol plus mild to moderate strength opioids) as the next step. Powerful oral opiates such as morphine may be appropriate in carefully selected patients with non-malignant disease who have not shown a good response to milder analgesics. Stimulant laxatives will generally need to be used as well, given the common side-effect of constipation.

A suitable example would be MST Continus tablets, at an initial dose of 10–20 mg 12-hourly. Transdermal fentanyl may provide better pain relief, and seems to result in less constipation and nausea than oral morphine. Its main disadvantage lies in the fact that each skin patch is applied for 72 hours, so titration of the dosage is difficult.[10] Suitable patients can be commenced on a 25 micrograms/hour or 50 micrograms/hour patch. Short-acting opiates may be needed for breakthrough pain or breathlessness.

Non-steroidal anti-inflammatory drugs (NSAIDs) will be useful for dealing with bone or joint pain. Co-prescribing proton pump inhibitors can help to protect the gastric mucosa. Alternatively, the newer COX-2 agents can be used. Neuropathic pain may respond to tricyclic antidepressants in low or moderate dosage (e.g. amitriptyline initially 10 mg at night) or anticonvulsants (carabamazepine 100 mg increasing to 200 mg daily, or gabapentin increasing to 300 mg three times a day).

Dyspnoea

Breathlessness can be helped by oxygen and low-dose opiates. Oxygen can be provided in the form of cylinders, or by using oxygen concentrators. The latter are likely to require the co-operation of a specialist chest medicine team. The anxiety that usually accompanies dyspnoea may require treatment with anxiolytic or neuroleptic agents.

Gastrointestinal symptoms

Nausea can be helped by the familiar phenothiazines cyclizine or prochlorperazine. Both of these agents and haloperidol are also useful for relieving anxiety. Prokinetic drugs include metoclopramide and domperidone. The more costly serotonin antagonist anti-emetics should rarely be needed. Oral corticosteroids improve appetite in cancer patients, so may be worth considering in other conditions.

Confusion

Delirium is often not recognised in people with organic illness, but it causes much distress, especially to the patient's relatives. Low doses of haloperidol (1–2 mg 2–3 times daily) or chlorpromazine (up to 100 mg daily) are useful. Such medication does more than sedate the restless or agitated. There appears to be an underlying thought disorder, which is also found among the more quietly confused.[11]

Depression

Depression, like delirium, is common in terminal illness. Patients may become depressed because of delays or difficulties in making a diagnosis, or due to having an incurable illness with a prolonged course and multiple troublesome symptoms. Because doctors often fail to make the diagnosis of depression, much avoidable suffering results. However, it can be difficult to distinguish the usual 'biological features of major depression,' such as weakness and lack of motivation, from the symptoms of the underlying organic condition. Depression is likely to be the cause of early-morning waking not caused by pain or breathlessness. Useful additional clues include inappropriate feelings of guilt, hopelessness or worthlessness or suicidal ideation. One study suggests that simply asking 'Are you depressed?' will identify almost all dying people with significant mood disturbance.[11]

Tricyclic antidepressants may help chronic pain, but anticholinergic side-effects (e.g. dry mouth) are a disadvantage. Selective serotonin reuptake inhibitors (SSRIs) such as fluoxetine or citalopram are now widely used and may be better tolerated in individuals who are seriously ill with organic disease.

Nutrition

Advice on nutrition may be needed in cases of advanced cardiac failure or COPD, with nutritional supplements being useful for cachectic symptoms. In neurological diseases, dysphagia or chewing difficulties are common. Salivary dribbling will usually respond to an anticholinergic agent. Nasogastric tube feeding may be used, but this is not pleasant or well tolerated. Nutritional support using a percutaneous endoscopic gastrostomy tube has advantages.

Some authorities have pointed out that patients with advanced illness who stop drinking may not need artificial feeding or rehydration. The main symptom that results is a dry mouth, which responds to simple mouth care. Nasogastric or percutaneous gastric tubes are often inserted in patients who are aspirating, but they continue to aspirate after this procedure.[11]

For those who are able to take nutritional supplements orally, there is a wide variety available on prescription, and advice from a local dietitian may be necessary. Whichever option is chosen, where possible the patient should make the decision after the provision of appropriate information.

Multiple pathology: a holistic view

Many of the above diseases are common in old age, often in their milder forms. In the elderly, multiple pathology (probably with attendant polypharmacy) is of course the rule rather than the exception. The treating doctor will need to be careful that the treatment of one condition does not worsen another. The aim and intention of each treatment needs to be reconsidered when life expectancy is limited. If drugs are introduced to treat one symptom, then it may be appropriate to review the list of drugs to see what can be omitted.

Special considerations apply to the treatment of risk factors intended to reduce the likelihood of possible future events. It may be appropriate to continue hypotensive agents or antiplatelet medication to prevent stroke (often in reduced doses), but the use of statins to lower blood lipid levels seems unnecessary in patients who have reached the stage of treatment with opiates.

The place of treatment

Deficiencies in the existing care of patients with conditions such as heart failure and COPD include poor communication with professionals, and a lack of practical and emotional support. Such findings have led some authorities to suggest that palliative care clinicians should be more actively involved in the management of such patients. There are too many potential patients for this to become reality for more than a few, although hospice-type care may have an educational and practical demonstration role. Most patients will continue to be cared for in general hospital wards, in nursing and residential homes, or in their own homes. What is important is that the philosophy of palliative care that is attributed to the hospice movement is applied to all of those with progressive incurable diseases in order to improve their quality of life. Where symptom control is not achieved, involvement of a palliative medicine specialist is both appropriate and necessary.

Intermediate care

Palliative medicine overlaps the care of the elderly, as the latter includes both rehabilitation and palliation. The primary healthcare team will look after patients with advanced illness in their own homes, in nursing homes and in community hospitals.

Communicating with patients, relatives and other carers

Breaking bad news

There are a number of simple rules that are now widely applied when communicating bad news to patients.

1   Find a quiet, private setting in which to sit and talk with the patient face to face.
2   If possible, a partner or family member should accompany the patient.
3   Find out how much the patient wants to know about their condition.
4   Assess the patient's understanding of their disease so that the news is understood.
5   Give the bad news directly in straightforward language.
6   Listen and respond to the patient's reactions, and be alert for buried questions. Expect tears.
7   Provide information in small chunks; often the patient cannot absorb much more.
8   Demonstrate empathy.
9   Ask if the patient has any additional questions.
10   Be prepared for reactions of denial or anger.
11   Emphasise the availability of support, and explain how the patient can obtain it.
12   Ensure follow-up and plan for a further meeting soon. Suggest that they bring a list of questions to that meeting.

Sharing bad news: special features of non-malignant conditions

Non-malignant disease typically has a longer and more uncertain time course than cancer. For instance, the patient with COPD may have had symptoms for many years, or indeed may have suffered symptoms long before the diagnosis was made. Over time there may be a number of relapses and remissions. The patient may suffer disease flares, pulling back each time, but eventually succumbing. The doctor needs to be sensitive to requirements for more information or other guidance, which are often unspoken. Of course people vary with regard to the amount of information that they want, and this can change with time.

You could ask 'Are you the sort of person who likes to know all the details? Or do you prefer to leave everything to the doctors?'.

If the response is the latter, it may be sensible to ask again later on, when the patient may be more ready for a frank discussion. Check the patient's present degree of knowledge and understanding: 'What do you understand about heart failure?'.

If there are questions about the prognosis, the patient has probably formulated some idea of the length of life that they can expect: 'What are you thinking about how long you might have?'.

The prognosis is always difficult to estimate accurately, especially in non-malignant diseases. For instance, about 50% of patients with heart failure will die suddenly.

Recent qualitative research in New Zealand has illuminated the coping strategies adopted by heart failure patients, including avoidance, disavowal, denial and acceptance. Disavowal is a distinct mechanism whereby patients who basically understand the threat to their life situations seek hope by positively reconstructing this threat. Doctors can help to support a positive adjustment by the way in which they talk to patients, including the telling of useful stories.[12]

References

1 Lonn E and McKelvie R (2000) Regular review: drug treatment in heart failure. *BMJ.* **320**: 1188–92.
2 Gibbs LME, Addington-Hall J and Gibbs JSR (1998) Dying from heart failure: lessons from palliative care. *BMJ.* **317**: 961–2.
3 Rogers AE, Addington-Hall JM, Abery AJ *et al.* (2000) Knowledge and communication difficulties for patients with chronic heart failure: qualitative study. *BMJ.* **321**: 605–7.
4 Gore JM, Brophy CJ, and Greenstone MA (2000) How well do we care for patients with end-stage chronic obstructive pulmonary disease (COPD)? A comparison of palliative care and quality of life in COPD and lung cancer. *Thorax.* **55**: 1000–6.
5 Burns A, Dening T and Baldwin R (2001) Care of older people: mental health problems. *BMJ.* **322**: 789–91.
6 Grant A and De Cock K (2001) ABC of AIDS: HIV infection and AIDS in the developing world. *BMJ.* **322**: 1475–8.
7 Adler M (2001) ABC of AIDS: development of the epidemic. *BMJ.* **322**: 1226–9.
8 Wood C, Whittet S and Bradbeer C (1997) ABC of palliative care: HIV infection and AIDS. *BMJ.* **315**: 1433–43.
9 Smith G and Charlton R (2000) New-variant Creutzfeldt–Jakob disease. *Br J Gen Pract.* **50**: 611–12.
10 Allan L, Hays H, Jensen N-H *et al.* Randomised crossover trial of transdermal fentanyl and sustained-release oral morphine for treating chronic non-cancer pain. *BMJ.* **322**: 1154.
11 Billings JA (2000) Recent advances: palliative care *BMJ.* **321**: 555–8.
12 Buetow S, Goodyear-Smith F and Coster G (2001) Coping strategies in the self-management of chronic heart failure. *Fam Pract.* **18**: 117–22.

Further reading

• Jeffrey D (1995) Appropriate palliative care: when does it begin? *Eur J Cancer Care.* **4**: 122–6.

- Shannon CN and Baranowski AP (1997) Use of opioids in non-cancer pain. *Br J Hosp Med.* **58**: 459–63.
- McQuay H (2001) Opioids in chronic non-malignant pain. *BMJ.* **322**: 1134–5.

Acknowledgements

The author would like to thank Gary Smith, Research Assistant, The Surgery, Hampton-in-Arden, Solihull, who reviewed the literature in relation to AIDS and vCJD.

CHAPTER 9

Role of the primary healthcare team in palliative care

Wolfram Jatsch

The challenge

Given the choice, the majority of patients when faced with the diagnosis of a terminal illness will express the wish to stay in their own home for as long as they can and, if at all possible, will want to die at home.[1] People with a progressive incurable illness have unique physical, psychological, emotional, social and spiritual needs, and looking after them in the community is a challenge for all those involved in providing care.

In recent years there has been a shift towards a specialist palliative care approach, and most patients will eventually die in hospital or in a hospice.[2] However, most palliative care patients will still spend much of their remaining time at home.[3] Thus the care of the dying remains an essential role of the primary healthcare team (PHCT).[4] Such care should be implemented in a competent and structured way in order to guarantee that the patient remains comfortable and pain free, and that dignity is preserved throughout the illness.

The advantages of palliative care provided by the members of the primary healthcare team are as follows:

- continuity of care
- a holistic approach
- work in the familiar home environment.

The role of the specialist palliative care team is to advise the PHCT throughout the patient's illness, and to be invited to take over care should this no longer be possible in the community.

Teamwork and communication

When dealing with a progressive incurable illness, all members of the PHCT should feel responsible for the care of the dying member of their community. It is vital to show a high degree of flexibility and motivation and to be accessible to patients, relatives and carers at this extremely difficult time.

Routes of communication within the PHCT can sometimes be convoluted. In order to overcome barriers of communication, each member of the PHCT needs a clear understanding of their own roles and responsibilities as well as those of the other team members. The core elements of effective care of the dying in the community are good communication, sharing of knowledge and teamwork. In an ideal world, regular practice team meetings provide a platform for discussing patients, the progression of their illness and the effectiveness of treatment.

The following PHCT members should attend practice team meetings

- general practitioners
- GP registrar
- practice nurses
- district nurses
- specialist community palliative care nurse/Macmillan nurse
- practice manager
- practice receptionists
- health visitor
- community psychiatric nurse.

The general practitioner (GP)

Ultimate responsibility for the overall care and co-ordination of care of a terminally ill patient in the community rests with the GP. He or she has the responsibility for prescribing, and is likely to have a good understanding of the patient's past and present social, psychological and medical circumstances. Often the doctor–patient relationship has a long history based on trust and years of attendance at the surgery.

The GP has a major role in the difficult task of breaking the bad news when cancer or another terminal condition has been diagnosed.

The most important personal qualities that are required when dealing with the emotions and grief of the perplexed patient and their family are as follows:

- empathy
- caring attitude
- good communication skills
- understanding of the patient's personality
- good relationships with the patient's family and carers.

The need for a management plan

The prospect of dying is extremely frightening for most people. Their expectations have to be managed realistically, and a clear management plan should be developed together with the patient and their family at an early stage, when the patient still has the capacity to make competent decisions.

The GP must closely follow the developments during terminal illness. It is of paramount importance to be available for distressed patients and their relatives during the last weeks or months of the patient's life.

Quality information

Modern primary care requires patients to be given clear information about the likely course of events during their last illness, such as life expectancy and quality of life, the availability of help for them and their family, and the various treatment options. Patients should be given the opportunity to express their wishes, and their autonomy must be respected. Only fully informed patients can make valid choices.

However, it is important to remember that to preserve the patient's hope is one of the most valued key elements of good palliative care.[5] There is an art to giving quality information to the dying patient without depriving them of hope. This could be described as sincere controlled optimism that overcomes the desperate search for and possible implementation of futile treatment options. The GP must understand how much information patients and their families really want, and should tailor this to the individual's need for knowledge at a pace that allows them to cope.

All patients and their families should be given the following essential information:

- how to contact the PHCT members during the day
- how to access medical help out of hours and over weekends
- on-call arrangements and emergency telephone numbers
- the importance of good symptom control round the clock
- how to increase or modify self-administered medication
- symptoms of clinical deterioration and when to seek help
- how to recognise an emergency
- how to signal when carers can no longer cope.

Some GPs may even offer their home telephone or mobile number to patients in case they are needed:

- as a doctor familiar with their case
- as someone to give advice
- for emergency situations.

The GP as co-ordinator of care

Within the PHCT, the GP has a central position in orchestrating the palliative care of a dying patient in the community. Although his or her skills are not comparable to those of a palliative medicine specialist, on average every GP will see and look after five terminally ill patients each year. Basic knowledge of first-line symptom control is a necessary part of the repertoire of any GP, but it is also essential for them to understand their limitations in terms of both palliative care skills and time constraints. A joint domiciliary visit with a palliative care specialist and a Macmillan nurse can therefore help to outline a clear management plan if, for example, there are complex symptom control issues.

The GP is the gatekeeper, supervisor and facilitator of care. Much work can be delegated to other members of the PHCT and to secondary care agencies if necessary. It is eventually up to the GP in conjunction with the patient and relatives to decide when a patient requires admission to a hospital or a hospice.

The role of the GP includes the following:

- co-ordination of care
- availability
- regular review
- anticipation and prevention of crises.

The district nurse

The district nurse has a key role in delivering day-to-day nursing care and practical advice during terminal illness. Normally they are experienced nurses who are employed by the health authority. They do not work for one GP surgery alone but for various surgeries in the community, usually during the daytime. In order to be able to work and communicate effectively they should regularly attend practice team meetings, have a mobile phone and if possible call at a surgery daily to update the GPs or vice versa. The district nurse can visit patients in their homes at regular intervals or flexibly up to several times a day if this is felt to be necessary.

The various tasks of the district nurse in caring for the dying include the following:

- provision of emotional support
- building up good relationships
- 'hands-on' nursing care (e.g. pressure area care, wound dressing, bowel care)
- teaching relatives and informal carers the basic principles of nursing care
- supervision or administration of medication
- setting up of syringe drivers
- recognition of practical problems in day-to-day care
- identification of clinical or mental deterioration of the patient
- anticipating that a carer is not coping
- liaison work with the PHCT and other healthcare professionals.

The district nurse is in an ideal position to develop an understanding of the home circumstances and to assess the needs of the terminally ill patient, who may suddenly become very dependent. Simply getting into the bath or going upstairs may now seem like insurmountable tasks.

The needs assessment

Examples of what a palliative care patient may need include the following:

- splints
- commode
- wheelchair
- pressure mattress
- incontinence pads
- hosiery
- medical equipment (e.g. catheters, nebulisers, syringe drivers)
- home modifications to doors, bath and stairs.

The findings of the needs assessment should be discussed with the GP. A referral to Social Services and occupational therapy services may be necessary to provide the necessary equipment.

Box 9.1 Occupational therapists

Once the patient's needs are established, community occupational therapists can be asked to arrange home modifications (e.g. hand rails, stair lifts, bath seats) and provide necessary medical appliances to maximise safe and independent living. Occupational therapists will also give practical advice on practical problems and coping skills for both the patient and his or her family.

The district nurse as 'networker'

The district nurse is in a central position to liaise and 'network' with all of the other PHCT members. For example, information about increasing breakthrough pain, nausea or vomiting can be fed back to the GP, mental problems of patients and their relatives can be referred to counsellors and community psychiatric nurses, and financial and social issues can be referred to Social Services.

The district nurse's 'network' activities may even extend beyond the remit of traditional primary care. Manicure, hairdressing, aromatherapy, reflexology and massage are examples of services that are sometimes requested by dying patients, and they can give comfort, dignity and hope. An experienced district nurse will provide information and establish contacts with such service providers.

Caring for the carer

It is important to observe the changing pattern of the concerns and anxieties of the patient and their family and to anticipate when carers (who by definition are available to care 24 hours a day) cannot cope any longer, thus preventing their breakdown. Through his or her experience and the close family contacts, the district nurse is ideally placed to support carers and to recognise increasing psychological distress, especially if the family provides most of the day-to-day care for the patient. Admission for respite care or additional nursing care (e.g. Hospice-at-Home nurses, Marie Curie night-sitters) could be arranged to provide some relief for the mentally and physically exhausted carer.

After death

Another important task for the GP and district nurse is to visit the family after the patient has died. This usually involves bereavement visits after the funeral to make an assessment and provide support. If necessary and desired, the relatives may be referred for bereavement counselling.

Box 9.2 Funeral directors

Funeral directors (undertakers) help bereaved relatives to deal with death. They are professionally trained to counsel the bereaved during the period of mourning and to alleviate stress. They collect the body of the deceased and store it in the mortuary or the Chapel of Rest for viewing by relatives and friends prior to the funeral.

Apart from arranging the funeral, they will also support the bereaved with necessary tasks such as insertion of obituary notices in the press, floral arrangements, and contacting relatives, friends or the local clergy for spiritual advice. Relatives will be advised on the requirements of death registration, and if a cremation is required, the undertakers will contact the doctor who issued the death certificate for completion of the cremation form.

The specialist palliative care community nurse (e.g. Macmillan nurse)

These nurses are often Macmillan nurses, named after the charity that provides their specialist training through which they acquire special skills in palliative nursing and symptom control. They are not classically part of the PHCT, since they are usually employed by a hospice, where they can be contacted. However, many of these nurses have a background of district nurse training and they work in the community alongside the PHCT. Patients are referred to them by the GP, district nurse, palliative care doctors or hospital nurses.

The role of the specialist palliative care community nurse includes the following:

- visiting terminally ill patients in their homes
- advising the PHCT, patients and relatives

- passing on their specialist knowledge
- performing specialist palliative care needs assessments
- arranging and facilitating day care and respite admissions to the hospice
- providing bereavement support
- link work with secondary care.

Through their specialist training, specialist palliative care community nurses are able to advise the GP on palliative medication and thus influence prescribing. However, they will not normally be involved in 'hands-on' nursing and out-of-hours care.

The link with secondary care

Their close contact with both the primary healthcare team and the hospice gives the Macmillan nurses a unique role as advisers and support providers for the terminally ill in the community. They can act as a link between the primary and secondary/specialist care level. Thus they are in an ideal position to approach palliative care specialists for advice on case management as well as referring patients to other specialist nursing services which are usually based in secondary care (e.g. lymphoedema nurses, breast and stoma care nurses or even oncology nurses, should special advice on aspects of radiotherapy or chemotherapy be required).

Box 9.3   The dietitian

Cancer patients tend to have an altered metabolism, nausea and suppressed appetite leading to cachexia and eventually food refusal. This often raises conflicts with the carers, who do not want their relative to die from malnutrition.

Dietitians may be asked by the PHCT to make a home assessment. They give advice on nutritional interventions such as appropriate caloric intake, liquidised food, high-energy food supplements and vitamin preparations. This ensures that everything possible is done to counteract physical decline and to preserve a basic quality of life.

The practice nurse

The practice nurse's main role is in supporting palliative care patients within the GP surgery where she is employed, although occasionally she may visit patients at home. A practice nurse often knows patients with a progressive incurable illness very well, and will share her knowledge of lifestyle, diet and coping strategies with these patients, as well as providing emotional support. Wound and pressure sore care, venepuncture and blood pressure monitoring are part of her involvement with palliative care patients. More recently, practice nurses have been given limited power to prescribe.

Although there is some overlap of her role with the district nurse's work, the practice nurse may not have the same amount of first-line patient contact, particularly towards the end of a terminal illness when patients are less able to attend the surgery.

The practice receptionist

Receptionists are trained to understand the subtle differences between those who demand a service geared to their own individual requirements and those who are in acute need. Palliative care patients are extremely vulnerable to physical and psychological distress, and should have priority over most other patients. The receptionist's role is to identify and communicate this quickly and efficiently to those PHCT members who are most likely to be able to help.

Receptionists are important for the following reasons.

- They will often have known patients and their families for years.
- They work closely with healthcare professionals.
- They are good listeners.
- They know 'what's going on' in the practice and their community through overhearing conversations and passing comments.
- They are sensitive to genuine calls for help.

Hospice-at-Home nurses

Like the Macmillan nurses, Hospice-at-Home nurses are qualified palliative care nurses. They are based in the hospice but practise in the community. They normally work during the daytime, and patients can be referred to them by the PHCT or by Macmillan nurses. Hospice-at-Home nurses have a new emerging role and as yet are not widely available throughout the UK.

The new concept of Hospice-at-Home nurses can be summarised as follows.

- They have experience in palliative care nursing.
- Their skill mix is comparable to that of a Macmillan nurse, with a strong emphasis on practical nursing care.
- They provide 'hands-on' nursing care for patients in their homes.
- They can provide more extensive nursing time than the district nurse.
- They may enable the patient to avoid hospital or hospice admission if this is desired by the patient and their family.
- Very ill and dependent patients or those who have no informal carer should be their main focus of activity.

In areas where district nurses are very busy and the service is over-stretched, Hospice-at-Home-nurses have an important role. However, their caseload has to be limited to enable them to provide good care. Ideally they should work very closely with the district nurse, and their time should be well organised to prevent overlap of nursing care provision.

Marie Curie nurses

These nurses provide a night-sitting service, which is widely available throughout the UK. The local service is usually contacted by the district nurse or the GP. Marie Curie nurses are registered general nurses, enrolled nurses or nursing auxiliaries. They receive induction training before working with patients, as well as continuing education in palliative care nursing. Their individual grade of skill is usually matched to patients' requirements and consists of 'hands-on' nursing care.

Box 9.4   The Marie Curie charity

The Marie Curie nurses are funded by this charity and complement the district nurse service, mainly at night and sometimes during the day, free of any charge. The service can reach up to 50% of cancer patients who are cared for at home in the UK. The aim of the service is to give informal carers the opportunity to have some time for themselves to rest and relax as well as to do the housework, shopping and other necessary daily tasks.

The community pharmacist

Palliative care patients are often on numerous drugs with complex side-effect profiles and rapid tolerance development. Community pharmacists and dispensers employed by rural dispensing practices have a wealth of expertise to share with the PHCT through their knowledge of drugs used for palliation and pharmaco-dynamics. Since GPs are not experts in palliative medicine, they may need to be advised by pharmacists on new drug formulations or alternative treatment regimes which are otherwise rarely used in primary care.

The pharmacist's role in helping the terminally ill includes the following:

- helping patients and relatives to understand the nature of their medication
- explaining the prescriptions given to them by their doctor
- giving advice on how more complicated systems of drug delivery (e.g. syringe drivers or slow-release adhesive patches) can be used safely
- supplying compliance aids (e.g. pill dispensers, medi-wheel) which help patients to take their medication exactly as prescribed (these aids are not available on prescription).

A better understanding of the purpose of a medication, how to take it and how to recognise any adverse side-effects will help to maximise patient compliance and thus achieve better symptom control.

The physiotherapist

Community physiotherapists are now more widely available, and members of the PHCT are increasingly able to refer patients to them directly, thus avoiding lengthy hospital waiting-lists. This is of particular importance when dealing with the terminally ill whose life expectancy is limited. Most community physiotherapists have had training in symptom control in palliative care patients, and will visit patients in their own homes if necessary.

Physiotherapists can help palliative care patients in the following ways:

• performing chest and lymphoedema drainage
• treatment of neuropathic pain (e.g. with transcutaneous nerve stimulation, TENS)
• giving patients exercises which aim to improve muscle strength and balance
• helping patients to stay mobile and strong for as long as possible
• giving advice on posture and lifting
• providing walking aids.

Factors that lead to cancer-induced immobility include bony and neurological metastases, metabolic complications, cachexia and pain. Palliative physiotherapy aims to help patients to lead as normal a life as possible in the face of diminishing resources. To be able to do as much as possible is a very important factor in preserving a patient's dignity during the phase of life leading up to death.

The social worker

The PHCT and Social Services have traditionally close working relationships, but referrals will be accepted from any source, including the patient him- or herself. Social workers must have a qualification in social work, and are employed by the local council.

Palliative care patients who are referred to the Social Work Department will receive a detailed needs, risk and financial assessment by the responsible care manager. This assessment includes issues of physical and psychological vulnerability as well as personal relationships, personal care, hygiene, medication and nutritional needs. When the data have been collated and discussed with the PHCT, a so-called 'package of care' is developed if the patient wishes to stay at home during their final illness.

Social Services social workers can arrange the following:

• meals on wheels at low cost
• home helps to do the patient's housework, shopping and laundry, and to collect prescriptions
• day care in local residential or nursing institutions
• emergency alarm systems

- home assessment by occupational therapists
- advice to patients about benefits.

Box 9.5   The special rules of terminal illness

For patients with a terminal prognosis of less than six months there is a fast-track system to an Attendance Allowance (AA) to support home care. For quick processing, the GP has to complete a standard form (DS 1500) and send it to the local Benefits Agency office for approval as soon as a terminal illness is diagnosed, together with completed section 1 of an Attendance Allowance Form.

The counsellor

Although requirements vary, most community and practice counsellors will have a recognised qualification or sometimes even a special palliative care counselling qualification, which is offered at various universities throughout the UK.

Counsellors can help patients and their families to cope with terminal illness in the following ways.

- They can see patients and relatives at regular intervals.
- They have an understanding of the effect that life-threatening illness has on relationships, and of the experience of bereavement.
- They know the issues that are raised by death and dying.
- They mainly use reflection as a tool for the resolution of these complex issues.
- Their approach is patient centred and has to be delivered in a sensitive and confidential way for it to be successful.
- They may cross-refer to specialist bereavement counsellors those bereaved relatives who show abnormal bereavement reactions or inability to adjust.

Box 9.6   CRUSE

This is a registered national bereavement charity. Local branches of CRUSE provide bereavement counselling by trained volunteers, a befriending service, home visits and social meetings. Bereavement is associated with a high mortality, and up to one-third of bereaved people develop a depressive illness. The strain of caring for a terminally ill person for longer than six months is associated with poor outcome. Counselling should be targeted in particular at these individuals, and at those who perceive their social support to be lacking or unhelpful.[6]

The community psychiatric nurse

Community psychiatric nurses (CPNs) have extended psychiatric nursing training and are concerned with the patient in a social context. Palliative care patients are sometimes referred to them by the GP for an assessment of depression.

It is a very difficult task to diagnose depression in palliative care patients. Sadness and despair are a recognised part of severe physical illness, especially when this is irreversible. Hence understandable dysphoria is not the same as depression which can be treated. Moreover, lethargy, loss of interest and anorexia may be caused by the terminal illness of the patient rather than by depression. On the other hand, deeply depressed palliative care patients may respond positively to humour, good news and tender loving care.

In order to clarify this often confusing picture, a CPN may be asked by the GP to perform an in-depth mental state examination, if necessary on the basis of repeated visits. While there may not be scope for a future-orientated and positively directional approach, the medical treatment of depression remains an important part of the overall management. The probability of depression should be discussed with the GP, and the prescription of an antidepressant, which may also be used as a co-analgesic, may be justified. The need for a sedative, anxiolytic or hypnotic is another area which may be explored by the CPN.

References

1 Townsend J, Frank AO, Fremont D, Dyer S, Karin O and Algarve A (1990) Terminal cancer care and preference for a place of death. *BMJ*. **301**: 415–17.

2 Higginson IJ, Astin P and Dolan S (1998) Where do cancer patients die? Ten-year trends in the place of death of cancer patients in England. *Palliative Med*. **12**: 353–63.

3 Seale C and Cartwright A (1994) *The Year Before Death*. Avebury, Aldershot.

4 Doyle D (1998) *The Way Forward – Policy and Practice. National Council for Hospice and Specialist Palliative Care Services. Report of a joint conference promoting partnership, planning and managing community palliative care*. National Association of Health Authorities and Trusts and National Council for Hospice and Specialist Palliative Care Services, London.

5 Leydon G, Boulton M, Mynihan C *et al*. (2000) Cancer patients' information needs and information-seeking behaviour: in-depth interview study. *BMJ*. **320**: 909–13.

6 Sheldon F (1998) ABC of palliative care. *BMJ*. **316**: 456–8.

CHAPTER 10

The plight of the informal carer

Jo Piercy

What is an informal carer?

Informal carers are people who have accepted the main responsibility for providing care for someone close to them. That person, due to illness, disability or frailty, is unable to manage at home independently and requires frequent or constant attendance.

Informal carers, whom we shall refer to as carers, are most often spouses, partners or other family members, but may also be neighbours or friends of the patient. The general household surveys of 1985 and 1990 revealed that there were up to 6 million carers in the UK providing varying degrees of care. Nearly 1 million of them were providing at least 50 hours of care per week.

Characteristics of carers

- They are most commonly female.
- They span all social classes.
- They span all age groups. The peak age for caring is in the fifth to seventh decades of life.[1]
- Many older people are carers. Over 33% of informal care for people over 65 years of age is provided by people over 70 years of age.[1]
- Among cancer patients, 33% receive care solely from one close relative, and half are cared for by two or three relatives – typically a spouse and an adult child.[2]

Without this support from family and friends it would be impossible for many patients to remain at home.

A job 24 hours a day

Carers are often providing round-the-clock supervision. They report the feeling of being 'constantly on call.' Their role is diverse. Intimate tasks are frequently performed, including washing, dressing, toileting and feeding. More physical demands may include lifting or transferring the patient from bed to chair. Some carers may be required to change dressings or administer drugs (i.e. basic nursing skills). This is an area where the informal carer is generally inexperienced and requires training, equipment and professional advice.

Carers are involved in the care plan for the patient. This will involve contacts with different members of the primary healthcare team (PHCT), together with attendance at hospital outpatient departments.

In addition to the above, carers still need to 'run the house' and carry out the many necessary daily chores (e.g. cooking, shopping, washing and housework). They will also be responsible for financial matters. Many carers will be continuing to work part- or full-time, or otherwise will be managing on a reduced income.

Caring is a daunting task. As a result of the difficulties and challenges that face carers, they often have no time left for themselves. It is very important to preserve this personal time, and it helps to reduce stress. Here follows some simple advice to try to assist carers who are coping with the burden of providing 24-hour care.

- Take one thing at a time.
- Look after yourself – get some sleep, and take regular meals and exercise.
- Take a break – do something you really enjoy.
- Try to relax – listen to music, practise meditation, etc.
- Join a local support group.

Loneliness

The role of the informal carer is highly idealised by society. Images are evoked of self-sacrifice, infinite patience and understanding. This inhibits carers from revealing their true emotions or needs, as they feel it is unacceptable to do so. They feel that any thoughts for themselves show them to be self-centred and inadequate.

This situation is not helped by healthcare professionals, who often do not think to ask after the carer's own well-being. In the words of one carer:

> I feel abandoned by a healthcare system that commits resources and rewards to rescuing the injured and ill, but then consigns such patients and their families to the black hole of chronic care.[3]

Informal carers will have contact with the PHCT on certain predictable occasions, including the following:

- at the time of diagnosis
- when the patient's condition changes
- when the carer becomes ill
- when the carer requires more information about the patient's prognosis or condition
- when the patient is transferred to institutionalised care
- when the patient dies.

It is essential that all members of the practice staff recognise these contacts as opportunities to improve their understanding of the carer's feelings, and develop some strategies for responding to them.

When feelings are expressed by carers, they include resentment, confusion, loss, helplessness, embarrassment and feeling trapped. Anger and guilt are common emotions, together with feelings of anxiety or being 'out of control.' One of the most difficult aspects is standing by and watching their loved one deteriorate.

Carers are often afraid. They fear the unknown if they have received inadequate information about what to expect. They worry about leaving their relative alone with others. They are also concerned about how to manage the patient and themselves during the final hours of death. However, these fears are not usually addressed.

Due to the huge demands that are placed upon them, these people neglect their own health and have no time left for continuing hobbies or socialising. Moreover, they have no time for other family or friends. As local family structures change, this exacerbates the problem. The result is an overwhelming sense of isolation.

Who cares for the carers?

In 1999, the NHS Executive published a White Paper entitled *Caring About Carers: a National Strategy for Carers.* This document describes the difficulties that carers face, and emphasises that carers should be treated as partners in the process of care with needs of their own:

> We intend to make progress so that more carers – and eventually all carers – feel adequately prepared and equipped to care if that is what they choose to do, feel cared for themselves, and feel their needs are understood.

Therefore primary care groups and trusts need to consider how their constituent practices might be more responsive to carers' needs and become more aware of the help that carers provide.

Ways to identify carers include the following.

- *Posters.* These could be displayed in the waiting or consulting rooms, encouraging carers to come and discuss their needs.
- *GP.* Awareness of carer strain needs to increase, but more importantly GPs should be on the lookout for it. Routine home visits might be indicated. Depressive symptoms should be sought, as they are treatable. GPs also have a pivotal role in co-ordinating services.
- *District nurse.* He or she will often know the home situation very well, and is in an ideal position to identify problems.
- *Receptionists.* They may also have knowledge of people caring for others in the community.

- *Computer search.* A search for all patients with certain conditions (e.g. multiple sclerosis or terminal cancer) will reveal the patient population and make it possible to identify the likely carers.

One of the best means of support is a local carers support group. Being among people who relate to the same situation prevents isolation and allows vocalisation of feelings. Members of the group care for each other and share emotions, which generates understanding and companionship.

Information on local support groups should be available from the GP practice, Social Services or the Carers Line (*see* page 149 for more details).

Needs of the carer

Traditionally the carer's needs have been given low priority by healthcare professionals. More than 50% of informal carers find the caring rewarding, 10% find it a burden, and the rest find it rewarding and burdensome in equal measure.[2]

The main needs of carers are outlined in Table 10.1.

Table 10.1 Main needs of carers

Need	*Comments*
Recognition	Carers want to be recognised for the value and importance of the work that they do
Be involved	One in three carers felt that their comments or concerns were not taken into account when arranging the patient's care plan[4]
Information	<ul><li>Carers require up-to-date information about sources of support or advice</li><li>Both patient and carer want to be able to make informed decisions regarding medical care. Being well informed reduces uncertainty and carer anxiety. The patient and carer need information on the importance of symptoms, prognosis and mode of death</li><li>Both patient and carer want to know how to seek help in an emergency</li></ul>
Support and training	<ul><li>*Practical support.* Education is needed on lifting and handling, and on drug administration and dressing changes. Carers generally have no nursing training and have to perform simple nursing procedures daily. In a survey conducted by the Carers National Association, 90% of respondents had received no advice on the above by NHS staff, resulting in high levels of anxiety.[4] Other practical help includes the provision of appropriate aids and appliances from occupational therapy services, and help with domestic support via Social Services</li></ul>

Table 10.1 Continued

Need	Comments
	• *Psychological support.* Around 46% of carers suffer from anxiety and 39% have depression.[2] Mild symptoms will improve with good communication skills by the healthcare team, but more severe symptoms will require recognition and treatment • *Social support.* This includes friends, family and local support group. Carers need time to themselves. A variety of different sitting services are available from voluntary organisations to enable carers to have time out • *Financial support.* Carers are often unaware of their entitlement to benefits. They may have given up work or decreased their working hours, resulting in reduced income. Social Services or the Citizens Advice Bureau should provide help with this. The local housing association may also assist with any essential repairs or improvements to the home • *Spiritual support.* Sitting services are available to permit carers to attend a place of worship
Confidant	Carers need to be heard and understood, and they need to be able to express how they are feeling. This role can be provided by a close family member or friend, or by the local carers support group
Coping strategies	Coping strategies can be divided into internal and external resources: • internal – faith, keeping busy, being positive • external – maintaining social networks, having people to talk to
Personal health	Carers need time out, time to sleep and time to socialise. They have complex emotional needs and commonly suffer from depression, poor concentration and sleep disorders. These problems frequently go unrecognised

The financial benefits that are available are frequently not claimed by carers, who may be unaware of their entitlements. A brief guide to the common benefits available is given below.

• *Invalid care allowance.* This is a benefit for carers of working age (16–65 years) who are spending at least 35 hours per week caring for someone who receives either the middle or highest rate of disability living allowance or attendance allowance. They must not earn more than £50 per week or be in full-time education, after deducting allowable expenses (National Insurance, pension, interest on savings).

- *Attendance allowance.* This is a benefit for people over 65 years of age who need help with personal care because of illness or disability. *It is not means tested.*
- *Disability living allowance.* This is similar to the above, but for people under 65 years of age who need care and also help in getting around. *It is not means tested.*
- *Income support. This benefit is means tested.* It is for people on low income.
- *Carers' premium.* This is not a benefit in itself, but an extra amount of money which is paid to a carer who is receiving income support, housing benefit or Council Tax benefit. The Citizens Advice Bureau can advise on who is eligible to receive it.

The role of respite care

Respite care provides a break for the informal carer. It often represents an essential coping mechanism, creating a little time for the carer him- or herself. It can be provided either in the home or in an institution. The service at home is predominantly provided by registered charities (e.g. Crossroads or Macmillan Cancer Relief). Local hospices have an important role in providing periods of respite by admitting the ill patient to the hospice for a variable length of stay.

Respite time must be arranged properly. It is important for the carer to know that their charge is safe and happy while they are not there. Respite care at home should be at a regular time, so that the carer can look forward to it.

Respite care can start from as little as 2 hours each week. The different types of respite care available are listed in Table 10.2.

Table 10.2   Types of breaks for carers

Night-sitting service	To allow the carer to get a full night's sleep
A sitting service	To allow the carer to visit family and friends
Daytime sitting service	To allow the carer to go shopping, etc.
Evening sitting service	To enable the carer to go out for a meal or go to the cinema, etc.
Inpatient care (e.g. hospice, residential care home)	To enable the carer to take a proper break and recharge his or her batteries. The patient can also receive a review of his or her needs
Day-centre attendance by patient	To give the carer a break and provide social contact for the patient
Holiday assistance	Some charities assist in providing holidays for the patient and their carer, either together or apart

When a carer can't cope: crises

Why now? What is the precipitating event?

A cause of the sudden inability to cope should be sought. Possibilities include the following:

- a change in the patient's condition (e.g. poor symptom control, general deterioration resulting in increased dependency)
- a problem with the psychological state of the carer (e.g. depression, exhaustion, anxiety)
- a problem with the physical state of the carer (e.g. illness of their own, severe insomnia)
- a psychological problem of the patient that makes the carer's life very hard.

What to do?

An urgent assessment of the situation is needed. Ideally this should adopt a multidisciplinary approach, but the initial assessment is most likely to be conducted by the district nurse or GP.

Discuss the various options with the carer – make sure that they are involved. Options include the following:

- additional voluntary help from family or friends
- respite care within the community
- respite care within a hospital or hospice, or residential care.

These crises often arise because, although the carer is aware that they are not coping, they do not know where to turn for help. Some suggestions are given below.

Where can a carer go for help?

- Contact your district nurse or GP.
- Contact your Macmillan nurse or hospice care team.
- Contact Social Services.
- Discuss your concerns with NHS Direct. Tel: 0845 4647.
- For general advice and support, contact the Carers Line (this service is run by the Carers National Association). Tel: 0808 808777.
- In a medical emergency, dial 999.

If the situation has not yet reached crisis point, some carers may find the following book helpful:

Health Education Authority (1994) *Caring: how to cope.* Health Education Authority, London.

This book is affordable and designed for both short- and long-term carers. There is an emphasis on feelings and ways of coping with them. It encourages attention to personal health and the continuing importance of valuing oneself. There are practical instructions on managing anger, relaxation techniques, back care and coping with depression.

Bereavement

Grief is the normal response to the loss of a loved person. In general practice the rates of consultation for both physical and emotional symptoms are increased about threefold in bereaved people for up to 6 months after their loss.

It is important for GPs and other members of the PHCT to have some understanding of typical grief in order to provide the necessary support and to recognise when the grief response is atypical.

Typical grief

Stage 1 – non-reaction
- This can last for anything from a few hours to up to 2 weeks. The bereaved person acts as if nothing has happened, and appears to be free from distress. In psychological terms it is a form of denial.
- Maintaining a 'public' face and organising the funeral provide distractions from reality.
- Emotional blunting, numbness and an inability to experience any emotion are frequent initial reactions.

After the realisation of death, a possible reaction supervenes.

Stage 2 – possible reaction
- The intensity diminishes within 1–4 weeks of onset and may be absent at 6 months.
- For several years afterwards, occasional brief recurrences are normal. They are often triggered by anniversaries, birthdays, etc.
- Psychological changes:

    (i)   depressed mood – guilt is very characteristic, and insomnia occurs in 80% of cases
    (ii) perceptual disturbances – a stranger may be fleetingly misidentified as a dead person, or noises may be interpreted as their voice
    (iii) preoccupation with memories that idealise and disregard faults of the deceased.

- Social changes:

    (i) withdrawal from social contact
    (ii) rejection of consolation
    (iii) resentment or open hostility.

- Physical symptoms:

    (i) autonomic reactions are the commonest such symptoms, lasting for 20 minutes to 1 hour each time. Symptoms include an empty feeling in the abdomen, breathlessness, and tightness of the throat
    (ii) other common symptoms include weight loss, blurred vision and regular headaches.

Atypical grief

- This is of greater duration and intensity than typical grief.
- Around 80–90% of cases are in women.
- The non-reaction stage persists for more than 2 weeks.
- The reaction can last for 2 years or longer.

Psychiatric illness

- This is six times more common in bereaved individuals during the first 6 months after the loss compared with non-bereaved individuals.
- Around 65% of cases have depression.
- Any psychiatric illness has a good prognosis in the bereaved and is unlikely to lead to chronic disability.

Mortality

- This is increased by sixfold in the bereaved person for one year.
- Spouses are most at risk, especially widowers.
- The cause of death is most commonly coronary thrombosis or arteriosclerotic disease.

Counselling

Most bereaved people do cope well. The main indication for help is when grief is abnormally severe or prolonged. Counselling can be provided by a variety of different members of the primary healthcare team, including doctors, district nurses, Macmillan nurses, social workers and psychologists. Trained counsellors are also available at the voluntary organisation called CRUSE – a service specifically designed for this purpose (*see* page 152).

Helpful information sources

Table 10.3   Useful telephone numbers

Carers Line	Run by the Carers National Association. Staffed from 10a.m.–midday and 2–4p.m. Monday to Friday. Provides advice and support to carers. Free information pack available. Can be difficult to get through, but is extremely helpful	**0808 8087777**
Carers National Association, UK office	Further advice for carers	**0207 4908818**
Disability Living Centre Helpline	A national information service that provides information and advice about equipment to help with daily living. Showrooms are also available	**0845 1309177**
Disability Benefits Helpline	General advice and information about benefits for people with disabilities and their carers	**0800 882200**
Disability Benefit Unit Helpline	Specific information on each individual's situation. Deals with Disability Living Allowance and Attendance Allowance	**08457 123456**
Invalid Care Allowance Helpline	Specific information on each individual's situation	**01253 856123**
Cancer Bacup	Nurse-led service that deals with questions relating to patient's condition	**0808 8001234**
Macmillan Cancer Relief	Information line to provide support for queries relating to diagnosis and the 'cancer journey'	**0845 6016161**
Crossroads Care	Service that provides trained care assistants to give carers a break. There are 207 schemes throughout the UK	**01788 573653**
Princess Royal Trust for Carers	General enquiry number to direct people to their local carer centres.	**0207 4807788 (UK)** **0141 221 5066 (Scotland)**
CRUSE Bereavement Care	Counselling services provided by trained counsellors *General enquiries* number will direct carer to their local branch *Bereavement line* is manned by trained counsellors 7 days a week (mid-afternoon and evenings)	 **0208 940 4818** **0845 758 5565**
NHS Direct	Advice on management of health problems	**0845 4647**

Useful websites

CRUSE; www.crusebereavementcare.org.uk

Disabled Living Centre (will answer emails as well as providing helful information): www.dls.org.uk

Carers National Association; www.carersuk.demon.co.uk

NHS Direct; www.nhsdirect.nhs.uk

References

1 Travers AF (1996) Caring for older people: carers. *BMJ.* **313**: 482–6.
2 Ramirez A, Addington-Hall J and Richards M (1998) ABC of palliative care: the carers. *BMJ.* **316**: 208–11.
3 Levine C (1999) The loneliness of the long-term care-giver. *NEJM.* **340**: 1587–90.
4 Wise J (1998) Carers are ignored by the NHS. *BMJ.* **316**: 1765.

Further reading

• Charlton R (1992) Palliative care in non-cancer patients and the neglected caregiver. *J Clin Epidemiol.* **45**: 1447–9.
• Charlton R (1992) The needs of informal carers during and following terminal illness in the UK and New Zealand. *NZ Fam Physician.* **19**: 167–9.
• Charlton R and Dolman E (1995) Bereavement: a protocol in primary care. *Br J Gen Pract.* **45**: 427–30.
• Charlton R, Sheahan K, Smith G and Campbell I (2001) Spousal bereavement – implications for health. *Fam Pract.* **18**: 614–18.
• Grbich C, Parker D and Maddocks I (2001) The emotions and coping strategies of caregivers of family members with a terminal cancer. *J Palliative Care.* **17**: 30–6.
• Murray-Parkes C (1993) Bereavement. In: D Doyle, GWC Hanks and N MacDonald (eds) *Oxford Textbook of Palliative Medicine.* Oxford University Press, Oxford.
• Simon C (2001) Informed carers and the primary care team. *Br J Gen Pract.* **51**: 920–3.
• Woof WR and Carter YH (1997) The grieving adult and the general practitioner: a literature review in two parts. Part 1. *Br J Gen Pract.* **47**: 443–8.
• Woof WR and Carter YH (1997) The grieving adult and the general practitioner: a literature review in two parts. Part 2. *Br J Gen Pract.* **47**: 509–14.
• Zisook S *et al.* (1994) The spectrum of depressive phenomena after spousal bereavement. *J Clin Psychiatry.* **55 (Supplement 4)**: 29–36.

CHAPTER 11

Spirituality and ethnicity

Barry Clark

Spirituality

'It makes you think, doesn't it?'. This comment was made by a patient in coronary care who was recovering from a heart attack. It was a simple recognition of a simple fact — we are all going to die. It is also a statement which opens the way to thoughts and conversations about our mortality and/or immortality. We are all going to die ... and then?

Most people build their lives around meaning. We work in order to have the means to play, and to pay our bills, and we retire to have the means to enjoy the fruits of our working lives. We raise our families and enjoy ourselves primarily in the context of this life and this world. To be faced with death is, for many, to be faced with the end of those traditional outlets for meaning, and to be faced with a future which is potentially meaningless. This is the territory of spirituality — connecting the 'here' with the 'there', the living with the dead, and meaning with meaninglessness. It is concerned with placing our own existence and extinction within the setting of the existence of the cosmos.

The patient quoted at the beginning of the chapter wanted to make it clear that for him any such thinking did not embrace the religious idea of a God or a Supreme Being, and this highlights the important relationship between religion and spirituality. Everyone can have a spirituality, whether it is sacred (e.g. Islamic) or secular (e.g. humanist), and some people choose to express their spirituality through religious beliefs and practices. However, choosing not to develop one's thinking about the relationship between existence and extinction along religious lines does not mean that spirituality is extinguished. The gap between meaning and meaninglessness still exists, and it is spirituality that bridges this gap. Often it is one of those areas that people are referring to when they talk of holistic or total patient care.

The potentially nebulous nature of spirituality may be one reason why we sometimes struggle in this area. In the era of evidence-based medicine and clinical governance, what are we to make of it?

> Spirituality in palliative care must contain sufficient dependable detail and description to enable it to be recognised, understood and studied — the surface of its reality and its knowledge — whilst we remain aware that this will not capture the intimate and inchoate — the depth of the reality and its more profound discernment.[1]

Models of the relationship between palliative care and spirituality have been developed,[2] but an equally important and related question concerns who delivers such care, and in the age of patient-focused care and multidisciplinary teams the simple answer is possibly the person who the patient asks. Therefore team members need to be aware of their own perspective and resources with regard to spiritual issues. 'It makes you think, doesn't it?' applies equally to patient and professional. If not, there is a danger that 'spiritual distress experienced by cancer patients may be under-addressed due to time constraints, lack of confidence in effectiveness and role uncertainty.'[3]

Ethnicity

The best advice one can offer here is to be aware of what a complex area this is. The most recent NHS national standard categories for the collection of ethnic information list no less than 17 categories (*see* Box 11.1), and are based upon a mixture of culture, language and family origin. It is not the same as nationality.

Box 11.1 Categories of the April 2001 NHS national standard categories for collection of ethnic information

White
British
Irish
Any other white background

Asian or Asian British
Indian
Pakistani
Bangladeshi
Any other Asian background

Other ethnic groups
Chinese
Any other ethnic group

Mixed
White and black Caribbean
White and black African
White and Asian
Any other mixed background

Black or black British
Caribbean
African
Any other black background

Not stated

If one looks at the principal languages/religions of the peoples of South Asia (i.e. Afghanistan, Bangladesh, Bhutan, India, Nepal and Pakistan), there are at least 12 languages and four religions (Buddhism, Hinduism, Islam and Sikhism). Culture is itself an amalgam of ideas, and Oliviere recognises that 'treating patients with cultural sensitivity involves all aspects of palliative care, from pain control to diet, and from modesty to bereavement rituals.'[4]

The problem of cultural stereotyping was highlighted by the report, *Opening Doors*,[5] and was confirmed and developed by Karim *et al.*, who showed that 'compared with white Europeans, there was an underutilization of day care and in-patient hospice services by members of the black/minority ethnic communities.'[6]

A good review of the cultural context of dying from cancer is that by Boyle.[7] This article highlights the need for knowledge and sensitivity, and offers practical guidelines and examples for assessing patients and their families.

Spiritual symptoms

> When I am dying, I am quite sure that the central issue for me will not be whether I am put on a ventilator, whether CPR is attempted when my heart stops, or whether I receive artificial feeding. Although each of these could be important, each will almost certainly be quite peripheral. Rather, my central concerns will be how to face my death and how best to help my family go on without me. A ventilator will not help me do these things — not unless all I need is a little more time to get the job done.[8]

While recognising the important diversity of definitions of spirituality and the even greater diversity of ethnic communities and their beliefs and practices, the above quote by Hardwig draws us to the fundamentally practical nature of our task when facing a terminally ill patient. Let us remember that, in this context, death within a limited time frame is no longer a possibility but more likely a probability, if not a certainty. The patient is looking for those who will accompany them and their family on that journey.

In healthcare practice we are used to gathering symptoms to enable us to develop a diagnosis and prognosis. Although these are often related to physical symptoms or social factors, the same idea can be applied to those symptoms that might be associated with signs of spiritual distress or desire.

- Why me?
- What have I done to deserve this?
- Am I going to die?
- Who will look after my family?
- How long have I got?
- Is there a God?
- I need to make my peace with the past/in the present/for the future.
- How will I be remembered?
- What about pain?
- I want to go/stay at home.
- I am so angry.
- I am so frightened.

Some of these symptoms require our practical skills and experience, which may lead to comparatively clear answers or suggestions, but others draw us into the realm of our own and the patient's belief systems. Although we may not be able to offer answers, and the patient often realises this as much as we do, it is important to acknowledge the questions and understand that this is often a time of unparalleled turmoil involving mixed and powerful emotions. I remember a nurse telling me how unfair it was that her mother had developed secondary growths from a cancer, and she raged against the God that she was not sure she believed in! She did not want her mum to suffer, but she was reluctant to call in the palliative care team because that meant 'the end.' She thanked me for listening and went away with no questions answered but aware that someone felt they were important questions.

The list of spiritual symptoms is by no mean exhaustive, and it must be considered in the light of the cultural/ethnic and religious background and practices of individuals and their families. In some traditions there may be a strong link between cultural and religious practices, but it is important to establish an individual's perspective in this area. You may pick up clues about a person's spirituality from their ethnic background and religion, but there is always the danger of stereotyping (e.g. 'All Asian families look after their sick and old'), so never assume, and always enquire.

However, it is worth recognising some of the central motifs within some of the world's major religions and relating them to some of the spiritual symptoms listed earlier. It must be emphasised that each religion has a variety of ways of expressing its faith, and it may be helpful at the appropriate time to ask the patient or their family which particular path within a faith tradition they follow.

Buddhism

Buddhism in its various forms is based on the life story of Siddhartha Gautuma, the Buddha or Enlightened One. The son of a wealthy king in North India, he eventually turned away from wealth after the Night of the Great Renunciation to seek his salvation.

Anatha (loss of self) is central to Buddhist philosophy. So much human energy is used to feed and sustain the ego (the self) when in fact it is an illusion and only temporary. There is an endless cycle of birth, death and rebirth, and suffering is part of this process. It is a person's Karma (every action has its consequences, either good or bad, and all bad actions must be compensated for) which goes from one life to the next. The ultimate goal is Nirvana – a timeless, deathless state.

As one's present life is ending it is better to think about the next one. It is felt to be important to retain a calm mind and not to dwell on one's earthly plans or family, as these may cause one distress or cloud the mind. With regard to pain relief, all pain has ultimately to be faced, if not in this life then in some other one. However, if pain is so severe that it impedes meditation, pain relief is appropriate not simply for the physical pain, but more importantly to enable the spiritual quest. We have to do whatever we can to allow the person to die in a calm, happy, peaceful state of mind.

Christianity

Like other religions, Christianity has a range of traditions within its fold. However, there is a central belief that Jesus Christ was the Son of God who died on the

Cross, thereby breaking the bonds of sin which separate humanity from God, and opening up the possibility of salvation for those who repent and turn to God. It is a resurrection faith that believes that after death there is a judgement to be faced, and one's eternal destiny (heaven or hell) depends on the verdict given.

There are many people who are only nominally Christian, and the struggle to believe can be as difficult as the struggle with illness. They may find it difficult to express their religious or spiritual beliefs, but are generally glad that there are those who can, especially as the illness progresses. Making peace with one's family, making peace with God by offering confession and receiving forgiveness and absolution, and making peace with oneself for past actions or omissions may be significant. The source of an illness may range from the simply 'lottery-of-life' approach to believing that the illness is specifically sent by God to test the person's faith, or sent by the Devil to try to break one's faith. Priests and ministers are often regarded as being at the vanguard for offering prayers and sacraments.

Hinduism

Hinduism is an umbrella term that covers a variety of beliefs, but one factor that unites them all is the belief that there is no absolute or exclusive truth. Another significant belief is that ideas are more important than facts, which only belong on the surface of things. Brahman is the only ultimate reality – the indescribable and formless 'ground of being'. It is a reincarnational faith and one's ultimate goal is to gain release from a separate existence and become one with Brahman. To achieve this one must break the chain of reincarnation (Samsara), and this possibility will be based on Karma (the balance of a person's deeds, good and bad). However, rather than being an upward and outward journey to attain spiritual harmony, it is a downward and inward journey to discover the nature of oneself.

If a Hindu patient is dying, their relatives may wish to bring in money and clothes for the patient to touch before distributing them to the needy. If the relatives cannot come to the patient, they may be grateful if staff can do this on their behalf.

Islam

The word Islam means 'submission', while the word Muslim means 'the one who submits'. This religion is based around the prophet Muhammad, who lived in the sixth century AD, and who received a series of revelations from the Archangel Gabriel, which were later gathered together to form the Qur'an. The five pillars of Islam are faith (Iman) in Allah and Muhammad as the apostle of God, prayer (Salat), giving alms (Zakat), fasting (Sawm) and pilgrimage (Haj).

Illness may be related to the will of God. This does not mean that Allah has willed it or is punishing the person who is ill, but it is the will of God in that had he willed to change it he could. Therefore it is quite legitimate to fight illness – 'For every illness there is a cure' (Hadith). One is expected to look for treatment, as the physical body is a gift from God, so even when dying we are to do what we can. However, whatever happens, 'Allah Akbah – God is great'. When one endures pain with patience there is a reward and sins are washed away. The suffering of the dying person is not in vain, but rather it is purifying. In general it is permitted to give whatever pain relief is necessary, although Islam does not accept euthanasia, and some patients may reject treatment because they feel that it clouds the mind.

Judaism

Jewish beliefs and practices are based on the first five books of the Hebrew Bible (the books of the law or Torah), but have been enriched and enhanced by the later teaching of the law, prophets and writings within the remainder of the Hebrew Bible, as well as the views of rabbis down the centuries.

According to Jewish tradition a person's life is measured by their deeds and whether they lived up to their potential. Therefore before death it is very important to review one's life, which may take the form of an ethical will. This is a statement to the family about what values the person wishes to pass on to the family – it is about philosophy rather than property. There is a strong strand which encourages Jews to fight against death, so much so that:

> the passion for life in Judaism is so great that to lose even a few minutes is thought to be a terrible thing. Indeed, all except three Jewish laws, the prohibitions against murder, idolatry and incest, may be broken in order to save a human life.[9]

As with Islam, euthanasia is not an option, but the hope is to die peacefully and enter Sheol (the Pit). Punishment and reward, including the idea of the resurrection of the dead, is not found in the Hebrew Bible. Life after death is when the soul returns to God – the natural end of all living things.

Sikhism

Sikhism has its origins in the fifteenth century AD when people in the Punjab became disaffected with their previous religions and became Sikhs (meaning disciples). Their leader was Guru Nanab, who sought to unite those who loved God and wanted to serve their fellow men. Fundamental to Sikh religion is the belief that God is one and man is made in the image of God. What a person does in this life will affect his or her soul, and evil intentions are rewarded by an endless cycle of birth and death. The reward for good deeds is to have this cycle broken. There is no great interest is the afterlife, since Sikhs can attain salvation in this life by devoting themselves to God and their fellow human beings.

Carers should be aware that those Sikhs who have chosen to 'take Amrit' will wish to retain, if at all possible, the five Ks (Kash – uncut hair; Kangha – wooden comb; Kara – iron wrist band; Kirpan – a short sword; Kach – short trousers/breeches). If these need to be disturbed or removed, this should be done with explanations and sensitivity. It is worth noting that there are no priests in Sikhism, so religious or spiritual needs may be met by any member of the Gurdwara. The latter is more than a place of worship. It is also the pastoral centre – the focal point of the Sikh community.

Euthanasia is not acceptable. The gurus regarded suffering as being a result of a person's karma. They must have the moral courage to bear suffering without lament and pray for the grace of God to endure with pain in a spirit of resignation and surrender. However, it is appropriate to relieve symptoms by medical and surgical means, as these are seen as instruments of God.

Practical spirituality

In the previous sections we have tried both to highlight the tremendous diversity of ethnic backgrounds and basic religious beliefs, and at the same time to identify some core spiritual symptoms that may apply. People who are diagnosed with a life-threatening illness enter a complex system where they may be described as follows:

- physically haywire
- mentally fragile
- emotionally unpredictable
- spiritually dynamic.

It is a time when theory is put to the test. Whatever their belief system, be it long established, recently discovered or newly hatched, it is now being put to the ultimate test. Will it bridge the gap between meaning and meaninglessness? The question is no longer 'How are you?' but more importantly 'Who are you?'. There may be a desperate need to re-establish the self or to nurture the damaged self. Those achievements and aspirations by which one identified oneself (e.g. career, ambitions, body image, relationships) are suddenly under threat. There is a need to make one's peace and to extract as much as possible from this life either as a preparation for death (extinction) or as a preparation for the next life (existential).

Spiritual pain

This draws us into the realm of spiritual pain. One of the major contributions of multidisciplinary teams is the management of physical symptoms, and apart from the obvious relief that this engenders, it also allows the patient to move to the more transcendent questions and to focus on and hopefully resolve issues of spiritual pain. Just as physical pain can separate people from their usual roles, so spiritual pain may separate them from their usual answers to life's ultimate questions as they wrestle with what *is* happening as opposed to what they believe *ought* to be happening.

What can we do, as healthcare professionals, to help to address these spiritual symptoms and the pain that they cause?

- Recognise the person, and not simply the patient. There is a need to affirm the individual and to find ways of determining their beliefs, hopes and fears. Address the person, not the disease.
- Listen to the patient's story and build up a picture. One of the problems is that we may not see someone until they are quite unwell. Encourage them to talk about their home/family/community/work. Do they have photographs? Time is often the greatest gift we can offer, and one of the advantages of primary care is that we may visit people in their homes and gain extra insights into the individual concerned.
- Recognise that while you may not share that person's spiritual or ethnic background, this does not prevent you from enabling them. What is required is the capacity to draw alongside another human being regardless of one's differences. What unites – that is, one human being's concern for another – has greater power than anything that might separate.
- Encourage, but do not enforce. One of the problems with illness is that it is like a rollercoaster. Once you are on it, you cannot get off! Autonomy is threatened, options are narrowed and personal space is challenged. Try to encourage the patient to recognise that while certain options may be more or less appropriate, choices are not necessarily right or wrong. People who are spiritually dynamic need space to explore.
- Emphasise the nature of the partnership between the patient, the healthcare team and the patient's chosen advocates (family/friends/religious community). Because illness cuts us off from our roots and our community, it is important that these links are re-established if possible.
- Be aware of your own spiritual journey. It may be unprofessional to extend one's personal pilgrimage into caring for others, but there is a need to be aware of one's own prejudices and biases, beliefs and doubts in order to prevent any snap judgements or prejudicial decisions.
- Be aware of your own limitations. One of the advantages of teamworking is the balance of strengths and weaknesses. The process of dying may raise profound questions to which there are no answers. It is important to share the burden with others and to pool resources.
- Be aware that spiritual care in primary care is not as focused and structured as that in hospital or hospice care. The danger is that it will simply get forgotten without chaplains, mawlana, priests, etc. to follow it up. This makes the task all the more important, and it should be documented.
- Develop your skills and knowledge. Some mosques, temples, Gudvaras, synagogues and churches have open days or open services to which all are invited, and many NHS trusts hold multicultural awareness training events.

We now live in a multicultural multi-faith society with significant communities drawn from a wide range of ethnic backgrounds. Although we may not be able to understand the diversity of beliefs and practices, we need to be aware that our professional role must be tailored towards finding a common meeting ground where our patient-focused care can be delivered with sensitivity and in such a way that the spiritual elements are given due recognition and respect.

References

1 Cobb M (2001) *The Dying Soul*. Open University Press, Buckingham.
2 Kellehear A (2000) Spirituality and palliative care: a model of needs. *Palliative Med.* **14**: 149–55.
3 Kristeller J, Zumbrun C and Schulling R (1999) 'I would if I could.' How oncology nurses address spiritual distress in cancer patients. *Psycho-oncology.* **8**: 451–9.
4 Oliviere D (1999) Culture and ethnicity. *Eur J Palliative Med.* **6**: 53–6.
5 Hill D and Penson D (1997) *Opening Doors*. National Council for Hospice and Specialist Palliative Care Services, London.
6 Karim K, Bailey M and Tunna K (2000) Non-white ethnicity and the provision of specialist palliative care services: factors affecting doctors' referral patterns. *Palliative Med.* **14**: 471–8.
7 Boyle D (1998) The cultural context of dying from cancer. *Int J Palliative Med.* **4**: 70–83.
8 Hardwig J (2000) *Hastings Center Report 2000, March–April. Spiritual issues at the end of life: a call for discussion.* Hasting-on-Hudson, New York.
9 Neuberger J (1999) Judaism and palliative care. *Eur J Palliative Med.* **6**: 166–8.

Further reading

• Aldridge D (2000) *Spirituality, Healing and Medicine: return to the silence*. Jessica Kingsley Publishers, London.
• Cobb M (2001) *The Dying Soul: spiritual care at the end of life*. Open University Press, Buckingham.
• Cobb M and Robshaw V (1998) *The Spiritual Challenge of Health Care*. Churchill Livingstone, London.
• Cooper J (ed.) (2000) *Stepping into Palliative Care*. Radcliffe Medical Press, Oxford.
• Murray Parkes C, Laungani P and Young W (eds) (1997) *Death and Bereavement Across Cultures*. Routledge, London.

CHAPTER 12

Ethics and dying

Derek Willis

Why ethics?

A recent television hospital-based drama series added a new member to its host of on-call characters. Not only was there an arrest team to call via a switchboard, but there was also an emergency ethicist. Presumably this was for those urgent ethical dilemmas that require specialist advice!

Perhaps we have not quite reached this situation yet, but it is certainly true that 'biomedical ethics' has flourished in an unprecedented way in the past 30 years. One could hardly have practised medicine in the UK in the recent past without being aware of the greater influence that ethics and law now have on clinical and research practice.

The term 'ethics' applied in these circumstances refers to a professional code of behaviour. It can be contrasted with a sense of personal morality, although the two may coincide. There may be circumstances where these two stances may cause difficulty for a practitioner. For example, a midwife may have religious reasons why she personally would not have an abortion. However, her professional ethics should mean that despite her personal feelings, she would still offer screening for fetal abnormalities to a pregnant mother. She would do this knowing that the results could persuade the mother to have a termination. What a practitioner feels or believes should not mean that a patient is barred from having all of the health options discussed and available.

Professional codes of behaviour are regularly questioned and challenged. The public's drive to understand their own health and to make choices in turn drives healthcare professionals to be more accountable for their actions and decisions. Doctors and nurses are now also questioning previously dearly held beliefs, particularly as medical technology makes them question not only whether they can but also whether they ought to intervene.

Ethics and palliative medicine

Palliative care may seem secure from such pressure, but the practitioner is often at the cutting edge of ethics at the end of life. The public as a whole is becoming more litigious in its outlook, and as such is more likely to challenge decisions that are made. The practitioner now has not only a moral duty to behave ethically, but also increasingly a legal one. Therefore it is important that practitioners have some understanding of the issues involved.

This chapter will initially examine some definitions, illustrating them with factitious cases, and will then apply these to palliative medicine. It is not possible to cover all aspects, particularly with regard to the law. The law changes so quickly that a book is often out of date as soon as it is printed. The aim of this account is to raise awareness, pose some questions and act as a stimulus for debate within primary care teams, and to stimulate further reading about this important subject.

Case study 12.1   Paternalism

Mrs Jones, who is 80 years old, has been admitted to hospital with a breast lump. She has had the breast lump for a couple of months but chose to tell nobody until it started to cause her pain and to discharge. The biopsy result shows definite carcinoma. The patient has not asked what the diagnosis is, as she doesn't like to bother the doctors. She would like to know what has been happening to her, but is too afraid of the doctors to ask. The medical team have not asked her whether she would like to know or not. The general practitioner and inpatient team have discussed her case and decided that she would not cope mentally or physically with any active intervention. They have also decided that it would be in her best interests if the diagnosis was kept from her. She is to be discharged from hospital tomorrow.

Medical ethics is classically described as having four fundamental pillars. These pillars, which can be used to weigh the merit of a particular medical action, are as follows:

- beneficence (always act for the patient's good)
- non-maleficence (never act to harm a patient)
- justice (evidence-based and fair action)
- autonomy (enabling informed consent).

The emphasis in practice has previously been to observe the first two of these principles. In summary, these two pillars state that medical practitioners should not actively harm their patients or do anything that would ultimately cause their distress.

These two principles are noble in themselves, but they can be used to justify medical staff making decisions for a patient without that patient's consent. It could be argued that this is the case in the scenario described with Mrs Jones. It is often felt that if patients know everything about their condition and treatment, they may give up. It is not fair, it is argued, to overwhelm patients with too much information that they do not have the capacity to understand. It is easy to see how this could lead to the underlying assumption that the 'doctor knows best'.

The term used to describe this situation is *medical paternalism*. A medical practitioner may feel that a particular treatment or action is in a patient's best interest. However, the doctor may not inform the patient of other treatment options that are available, as they may feel that they are better placed to make the decision than the patient. How could a person with no medical qualification make such decisions? Medical paternalism occurs when a medical practitioner makes a decision about a treatment that they regard as beneficial, without involving the patient in the decision and showing respect for the patient's autonomy.

It is easy to criticise such an attitude, but a practitioner who acts paternalistic-ally would argue that he or she is acting to alleviate a person's suffering. How-ever, ethics has undergone a change of emphasis during the past 30 years, and the autonomy of patients is now receiving more emphasis. Paternalism compromises a patient's decision-making capacity and is therefore regarded as undesirable. The patient should be allowed to choose which evidence-based action they feel is appropriate to their individual circumstances.

Paternalism can be summarised as follows.

- It does not give the patient choices.
- The medical staff are not acting to harm the patient.

Case study 12.2   Autonomy

Dave, the SHO in oncology, has nearly come to the end of his clerking list for the day's chemotherapy. He consents the penultimate patient of the day and gets his signature. It has become almost like clockwork now, as he has had to do it so many times. The patient asks how many more courses of chemo-therapy he is due to have and what the side-effects will be. Dave doesn't know the answers to these questions. Dave then discovers that his last patient is a retired Professor of Medicine and knows more about the chemotherapy than Dave does. The Professor of Medicine, who has bowel cancer, then explains the chemotherapy to Dave and also to the patient whom Dave consented earlier.

The term 'autonomy' is derived from the Greek phrase for a self-governing city. It is now used with regard to people and their ability to 'self-govern'. When used in a healthcare context, the principle of autonomy states that a patient has the right of access to the information that they need to make decisions regarding treatment options. This will allow a patient to make their own choices regarding their future care. Any human being should be allowed to make decisions on the basis of information and advice given to them by the healthcare professionals. This should lead to a situation of *informed consent*. In other words, a patient gives informed consent to a medical procedure when they have been given as much information as they feel is necessary for them to make that decision.

The problem with informed consent is that medical practitioners can be in danger of giving people too much information. If a patient is to be completely autono-mous, they must be allowed to decline information if they so wish. Often people feel that the idea of informed consent dictates that a health professional must tell everyone everything. Consultations would double in length if this were the case (e.g. general practitioners would read every side-effect for every drug that they prescribe to a patient). So long as the medical practitioner is not knowingly withholding information that the patient may need or want, then the patient is as fully informed as they need to be. It is therefore possible for a patient to know nothing, yet still to give informed consent. If this is the amount of information that the patient feels is appropriate, then informed consent has occurred. This is often a difficult balance to judge, and communication is the key to a good working practitioner–patient relationship.

Informed consent can be summarised as follows.

- It respects autonomy.
- It is not paternalistic.
- It allows the patient to decide how much information they want.

Case study 12.3   A 'good death'

Jenny, a hospice nurse, feels that she has failed. Two people have died tonight and their deaths were very different. Mrs Appleby was 90 years of age, had reached the end of her life and died peacefully with her family around her. John was 30 years old, had a young family and was very angry about his diagnosis. His death was loud, unfair, and he pushed his family away from him at the end. Jenny thinks that she has failed John and that he, unlike Mrs Appleby, did not have a good death.

So what relevance does all of this ethical theory have to palliative care? One of the recurring problems for practitioners who are involved in palliative care is defining what is meant by a good death. Is this an outcome that one can look back on, saying that a good death occurred and that this was a process in which healthcare professionals were involved? In an atmosphere of evidence-based medicine, how can practitioners show that a good death has occurred if it is unclear exactly what it is?

Perhaps a good death is what a patient says they wish to have. Practitioners may have their own ideas of what they would like to happen, but essentially it is not their death but that of the patient. People have different healthcare needs depending on their background, ethnicity, age and culture. Therefore one uniform idea of a good death will not fit all patients, and the concept needs to be tailored to individuals.

In this case study, the death of 30-year-old John was very different to that of Mrs Appleby. John may not have wished to have a calm accepting death. Mrs Appleby may feel that her death has not come soon enough and that she has done everything in her life that she wanted to do. Each could be defined as a good and appropriate death for the person concerned, although the deaths were very different. In that sense, Jenny the nurse did not fail either of the patients. It could be viewed as medical paternalism if someone says that they know what type of death is appropriate for a particular person. Only the patient knows what it is like to be them. The focus of care should be on providing the information and services to enable patients to have the type of death that is appropriate for them, rather than adopting a 'one size fits all' attitude.

This ethical focus challenges many aspects of care. If a patient makes an informed choice not to have chemotherapy, is it appropriate to persuade them to have such treatment? Conversely, if a patient makes an informed choice that they want chemotherapy which their palliative care team may feel will not have good results, should practitioners really actively seek to dissuade them? If a patient wishes to die at home, should the team not be trying to facilitate this? Holistic care focuses on the patient as a whole, and surely part of this involves empowering patients to make their own choices, thereby respecting their autonomy.

When does palliation start?

A question that is raised is the issue of when palliation starts. Sometimes medical practitioners are in danger of acting as if there is some cut-off point at which treatment definitely becomes palliative, 'when nothing more can be done'. This is often seen as a defeat or 'failure', when no more medical intervention can take place that is active and aimed at a cure.

However, if one defines palliation as the treatment of symptoms without curing the underlying disease process, is it possible to talk as confidently about an active/ palliative cut-off point? Much chemotherapy involves only a slowing of a disease process, rather than a definite cure. One cannot treat chronic obstructive pulmonary disease (COPD), but one can alleviate its symptoms. When does such treatment become palliation?

It could be argued that palliation is more gradual in its use in therapy than is often claimed to be the case. If this was communicated to the patient and medical staff, it could make withdrawal of active treatment easier to deal with when it has not been successful in achieving a cure.

Case study 12.4   Truth-telling

Mr Jones has lung metastases from his carcinoma of the prostate. You are due to go in to attend to him in the local hospital, but his daughter manages to halt you in the corridor before you go in. She asks you not to tell him about his cancer and how far it has spread. The family feels that he should not know and that he would not wish to know that he has cancer. You agree not to tell Mr Jones. You open the curtains for him and start to care for him. He looks you in the eye as you do this and asks you to tell him exactly what is going on.

The above scenario is a common situation for palliative care personnel – the so-called 'conspiracy of silence'. Relatives may not wish the practitioner to tell the patient their diagnosis or prognosis. A relative may feel that they are protecting their loved one from unnecessary distress by shielding them from the truth. If a patient asks about their diagnosis, what should one do in these circumstances? Whose wishes or requests should a practitioner respect the most?

Perhaps the issue at stake here is whose information and diagnosis is involved. If a patient asks a healthcare worker what is happening to them, then they surely wish to know the answer to that question. It could be argued that if a patient is asking a practitioner a direct question, then that practitioner is duty bound to answer the question as truthfully as he or she can. Trying to hide things from a patient who really does want to know what is happening to them is not only unethical, but also challenges the future relationship of the practitioner with that patient. If they were to find out that a practitioner had knowingly lied to them, why should they trust them again?

Perhaps in an effort to be holistic and to include the family in the patient's care (which in itself is no bad thing), the focus of attention for giving information has been on the family and not on the patient him- or herself. This approach is understandable, as it is the family who will be left at the end after the patient has died. Palliative care teams want to try to make the death as 'good' for the relatives and the patient as possible. One could also cynically assume that they often want to reduce the number of complaints that they receive! Once that patient has died, the staff may feel that they are open to criticism, as the patient is not around to defend them if they have acted against the relatives' wishes. However, if the palliative care team wishes to empower patients in their decision making, it should be the patient who decides how much information they want, when they want this information to be given to them, and who else they wish to receive this information. Where possible, and with the patient's permission, information should be given with the patient and their family present at the same time.

Case study 12.5 Advance directives

You have been the general practitioner for patient AH for many years. He infrequently visits you, but when he does come to see you, you feel that he is one of those people with whom you have a natural affinity. He sits down in the chair and puts a piece of paper on the table. It contains a lengthy description of what he would want done in the event of his becoming gravely ill. He wants your assurance that you will follow to the letter what is written on the piece of paper.

Advance directives (living wills) are a way in which patients can state categorically what they do and do not want to happen at the end of their life, should they not be in a position to state their wishes at that time. These can be legally recognised so long as the patient was competent at the time of writing them. The directive should also have been stated without any undue influence.

To perform an action without a patient's consent is recognised as 'battery' in law. Therefore if a directive were to be taken to court, it would be upheld as battery to the patient. This is reinforced in the Human Rights Act, but has the proviso that if medical science has advanced since the directive was written, then consideration of such medical advancement must be taken into account.

Advance directives do not have to be written, but the situation is much clearer if they are. It is easier to prove exactly what the patient has agreed to if it is formally set down, and confusion can be avoided. The author suggests that further advice should be sought when and if this situation arises. In addition, it may be appropriate for a patient to take legal advice to ensure that an advance directive is upheld should it be required in the future.

Case study 12.6   Doctrine of double effect

So far Edith has had no pain from her breast cancer, even though she has secondaries. You have received an urgent call to go and see her. She is in absolute agony and unable to get comfortable. You have no hesitation in giving her a small amount of subcutaneous diamorphine and starting a small amount of the same drug in a syringe driver. However, it does not seem to be working, and Mrs Jones is still in complete agony. Her daughter starts to express concern as you draw up some more painkiller. She asks if it is possible to give too much morphine to someone, and whether you could harm her mother with the drugs that you are giving her.

There are often situations where healthcare professionals may want to give a drug to a patient for their benefit, but they know that there may also be some potential form of harmful outcome. For example, a doctor may give a dose of opiate for pain relief that may prematurely shorten a patient's life. What is the legal and ethical situation in such circumstances?

A principle called the *doctrine of double effect* applies here. In this situation a person may plan to give a treatment where there are two possible outcomes – one good and one bad. For this to fit the doctrine, such a person must only intend the good outcome and not the bad one. They must also not gain the good outcome by the bad outcome occurring (e.g. achieving pain relief by the death of a patient). The good and bad effect must be in proportion to each other, and the good outcome must be something that is morally allowable.

For example, if a doctor were to give an opiate analgesic such as diamorphine to a patient, he or she must only desire a good outcome. In other words, he or she must only be intending to give the morphine to bring about pain relief. The risk of shortening the patient's life, it is argued, is in proportion to the need for pain control, and pain control *per se* is not immoral. They must not be intending to deliberately shorten a patient's life. If this happens, it must only be as an unintended consequence.

The case of Dr Cox [R. v. Cox (1992) 12 BLMR 12] illustrates this. A patient who had rheumatoid arthritis was given a lethal dose of potassium chloride because she was suffering from intractable pain. The doctor felt that everything that could have been done to treat this woman's pain had been done. The doctrine of double effect could not be applied in these circumstances, as there was no possible analgesic or therapeutic role for the drug. Potassium chloride was deliberately used to bring about this patient's death, and her death was the means by which her pain relief was achieved, rather than an unintended outcome.

Some would say that this doctrine is just splitting hairs, but there does seem to be a difference between deliberately bringing about someone's death and trying to provide adequate pain control. Patients must be given adequate pain control and information about its intended effects and possible side-effects, without healthcare staff fearing that they will be found to have been negligent. This should be written in the medical records, and if the patient permits it, communicated in the presence of a relative. The law recognises this with regard to certain medical treatments, so in specific circumstances the doctrine is legally as well as ethically recognised.

The doctrine of double effect can be summarised as follows.

- Only good is intended.
- Harm must be unintended.
- The harmful effect must not bring about the good effect.

Case study 12.7   Active euthanasia

Alice has asked for a home visit. She is housebound as she has been a long-term sufferer from multiple sclerosis. Visits to her house are always enjoyable, and you look forward to visiting her. Today she is different. She looks unhappy and tells you that she has really had enough. She feels that her life has reached the point where there is nothing in it that is worth living for. She asks you whether you agree with euthanasia and whether you would be willing to give her a fatal injection.

There are limits to a patient's autonomy. They may not request a medical practitioner to actively bring an end to their life, where the treatment given has no other aim but that end. Therefore a patient cannot autonomously decide that they wish their life to end, and expect a medical practitioner to fulfil this wish.

Euthanasia itself refers to the taking of a person's life by a medical practitioner as an intended intervention. The literal translation of the word is 'an easy death'. It is sometimes difficult to define exactly what would constitute an act of euthanasia. Many people would wish to draw a distinction between active and passive euthanasia. Active euthanasia is the giving of a treatment to directly cause the death of a patient, and legally this is regarded as murder. Thus in the case of Cox [R. v. Cox (1992) 12 BLMR], the active administration of potassium chloride constituted an act of active euthanasia.

Passive euthanasia

Passive euthanasia is said to occur when circumstances are created in which death can occur, rather than the death being actively caused. Thus in these circumstances a patient's life is ended by someone declining to perform a life-saving act or withholding treatment, rather than actively giving therapy to terminate their life. The concept of an omission of treatment and its distinction from an active killing was used to justify the stopping of artificial feeding in the Bland case [Airedale NHS Trust v. Bland (1993) 1 All ER 521]. Many people would not agree morally with the above distinction. For example, when can one say that an omission becomes an action? In an incurable disease, when should 'nature' be allowed to take its course?

Medical futility

Some people would wish to highlight the idea of medical futility and would argue that this is distinct from euthanasia. A practitioner does not have a duty of care to provide treatment that is deemed to be futile or that would prolong terrible suffering. This would not be for the patient's good. Thus the decision not to resuscitate patients with advanced cancer can be justified, as the illness is incurable, the resuscitation is unlikely to be successful, and it will probably result in a poor quality of life. Another example is the decision not to give antibiotics to someone with advanced cancer and a chest infection where it is felt that the infection will inevitably kill the patient despite the use of antibiotics. Many practitioners feel comfortable with this, as the patient's death is natural and not medically initiated. The choice lies in the intervention or non-intervention that occurs during that death. Thus death has not been caused by the healthcare team, and therefore it can be stated that euthanasia has not occurred. This discussion has further implications for how 'good deaths' come about.

On paper, the distinction between active and passive euthanasia seems simple, but it can be difficult in practice. Many people would also disagree about the definition of futility and the precise stage in an illness at which this is reached. Consider the following.

1   Patients can rely absolutely on the fact that a doctor will not perform an action that is intended to shorten their life. This is fundamental to the doctor–patient relationship. If euthanasia was to be made legal, it would weaken this trust and many patients might not feel that their doctor was always solely committed to their best interests.
2   Many authorities within the palliative care movement would argue that there is no need for euthanasia if correct and proper adequate palliative interventions are instigated to alleviate distressing symptoms such as pain.
3   Perhaps the push for euthanasia reflects our Western society's unease with death and the fact that it remains a taboo subject. Perhaps it is also a reflection of the fact that many people are worried about the possible level of intervention that healthcare staff can instigate. Palliative care teams should be at the

forefront of educating our society, re-establishing the fact that death is actually a part of living, not a medical error or 'failure'.

Conclusions

This chapter has described some of the issues involved in ethics at the end of life. Many of the issues have only been touched upon, and in no sense are any of the sections intended to be exhaustive. It is hoped that the reader realises that palliative care teams within the primary care setting cannot hide their heads and hope that such issues will not arise for them. It has already and will become more common for the primary care team to be involved in these ethical issues, especially as they are more likely than any other person involved in a patient's care to know their wishes. The references listed below should help the reader to develop a deeper understanding of the above issues.

Further reading

- Brazier M (1992) *Medicine, Patients and the Law* (2e). Penguin Books, Harmondsworth.
- Davies M (1998) *Textbook of Medical Law* (2e). Blackstone Press, Oxford.
- Gillon R (1994) *Philosophical Medical Ethics* (7e). John Wiley & Son Ltd, Chichester.
- Randall F and Downie RS (1999) *Palliative Care Ethics* (2e). Oxford University Press, Oxford.

Useful references

- Brook RH (1994) Appropriateness: the next frontier. *BMJ.* **308**: 218–19.
- Buckman R (1996) Editorial: talking to patients about cancer. *BMJ.* **313**: 699–700.
- Fallowfield L (1993) Giving sad and bad news. *Lancet.* **341**: 476–8.
- Finlay I (1994) Editorial: palliative medicine overtakes euthanasia. *Palliative Med.* **8**: 271–2.
- Franks A (1997) Breaking bad news and the challenge of communication. *Eur J Palliative Care.* **4**: 61–5.
- Girgis A and Sanson-Fisher RW (1995) Breaking bad news: consensus guidelines for medical practitioners (review). *J Clin Oncol.* **13**: 2449–56.
- Harrison A, Al-Saadi AMH, Al-Kaabi ASO *et al.* (1997) Should doctors inform terminally ill patients? The opinions of nationals and doctors in the United Arab Emirates. *J Med Ethics.* **23**: 101–7.
- Jeffrey D (1995) Appropriate palliative care: when does it begin? *Eur J Cancer Care.* **4**: 122–6.
- Killick J (1997) Communication – 'the truth is mine not yours'. *Scottish Med.* **16**: 4.

- McBride G (1994) Phase-one trials can exploit terminally ill patients. *BMJ.* **308**: 679–80; http://bmj.com/cgi/content/full/308/6930/679
- Merriman L, Perez DJ, McGee R and Campbell AV (1997) Receiving a diagnosis of cancer: the perceptions of patients. *NZ Med J.* **110**: 297–8.
- O'Neill J (1999) A peaceful death. *BMJ.* **319**: 327; http://bmj.com/cgi/content/full/319/7205/327
- Schneiderman LJ, Faber-Langendoen K and Jecker NS (1994) Beyond futility to an ethic of care. *Am J Med.* **96**: 110–4.
- Smith G (1995) Restructuring the principle of medical futility. *J Palliative Care.* **11**: 9–16.

CHAPTER 13

Thinking about bereavement

Alexandra Withnall

Introduction

Bereavement is one subject that most people probably prefer not to think about! In fact, until they are faced with it, most people have little idea of what to expect or how they should behave towards a relative, friend or colleague who has been bereaved. Of course, GPs and other members of the primary healthcare team will encounter death routinely in the course of their day-to-day work, but some medical and healthcare professionals may have had little training in understanding the different facets of bereavement or the aftercare of bereaved patients. Others may need to update their understanding of some of the physical and psychological effects that bereavement can have.

What do we mean by bereavement?

The word *bereavement* is derived from the root verb *reave*, which means 'to despoil, rob or forcibly deprive', so whatever the circumstances, bereavement implies some degree of individual *loss*. Of course, all of us experience a range of losses throughout our lives, and these can vary in nature from misplacing some favourite toy or object such as a security blanket in childhood, through events such as loss of a job due to redundancy, to the permanent loss through death of a beloved spouse, partner or other close relative at any stage of life. Some of the commonest types of loss are listed in Box 13.1.

Box 13.1 Examples of loss

Death of a spouse or close family member
Divorce or separation
Miscarriage/stillbirth
Death or loss of a family pet
Career or job change
Redundancy
Retirement

Moving house/entering residential care
Age-related changes in hearing/sight
Loss of mobility due to illness or disability
Loss of a body part through illness or accident
Being a victim of burglary or violence

In some cases, different types of loss may be linked. For example, redundancy may lead to an unwanted house move, or the onset of a physical disability may result from an act of violence. It is also obvious that some forms of loss may be sudden and life-transforming, while others may take place over a period of time or be fairly minor in nature. Occasionally, they may even have been welcomed at one level (e.g. moving from a house that has unhappy memories, or the ending of a disastrous relationship). However, regardless of the type and degree of seriousness of the loss, the immediate outcome will be as follows:

- *grief* – the individual psychological reaction to loss
- *mourning* – usually described as the process by which bereaved people cope with loss and grief through the cultural and social practices that pertain in their particular society or religion.

In practice, these distinctions may be rather too neat. It is more likely that grief and mourning are interconnected in that cultural beliefs may well affect the way in which people grieve as well as how they give expression to their loss.

Members of the primary healthcare team (PHCT) will inevitably come into contact with a wide range of different types of loss among patients, and it is important to remember that loss always involves some degree of *transition* and *change*. Some patients may have experienced multiple minor and major losses, while others may sail through life relatively unaffected until they are stopped in their tracks by what they perceive to be a sudden devastating loss. Since experiencing the death of a loved one is one of the most basic but also most painful aspects of human experience, we shall concentrate here on *bereavement as the loss of a relationship through death*, its aftermath, and the associated changes that a death brings.

Reflection Exercise 13.1

What kinds of losses have you suffered in your life so far? How did you deal with them?

The effects of bereavement

Recent years have seen a strong interest in the development of theory and research into bereavement and grief.[1] Early work on reactions to bereavement was mainly derived from Freudian traditions of psychoanalysis, but there have subsequently been a number of other psychological models of grieving following a bereavement. In particular, the notion that a bereaved person must pass through a series of psychological *stages* on the way to recovery, or that they must undertake a number of recovery *tasks*, although probably subject to misinterpretation over the years, has been particularly influential in the training of health and social care professionals and in the early development of bereavement care services.

Stages and tasks theories of grieving

Stage theories of dying and bereavement suggest that grieving is a *process* rather than a state. Sometimes referred to as 'grief work', these stages have been described in different ways by different authors. Probably the most influential work has been that of Parkes[2] and Kübler-Ross,[3] whose analysis initially related not to grief following bereavement, but to dying people's reactions to their own imminent death.

Box 13.2   Stages of grief

Parkes (1986)
Numbness
Pining
Disorganisation and despair
Recovery

Kübler-Ross (1969)
Denial
Anger
Bargaining
Depression
Acceptance

A second approach is to think in terms of the *tasks* of mourning that a bereaved person must undertake, rather than actual stages.

Box 13.3   Tasks of mourning (adapted from Worden[4])

To accept the reality of the loss
To work through the pain of grief
To adjust to the environment in which the deceased is missing
To let go of the deceased, to reinvest emotional energy in other relationships and to 'move on'

Therefore according to these types of models, the bereaved person must 'work through' grief and detach him- or herself from the deceased person. There is then thought to be a danger that the bereaved person will 'get stuck' at a particular stage or task and may suffer *pathological grief* (e.g. depression, anxiety disorders, somatic symptoms) which might require professional help.

How useful is the idea of stages and tasks?

Although the idea of tasks and stages has been so influential, it has been criticised on the following grounds.

- It suggests a definite pattern of 'healthy' grieving, which can be quite frightening for bereaved people who may be afraid that they are grieving 'wrongly'.

- It suggests that grief is time limited.
- It may lead people to assume that they can and should put the past behind them. This is an assumption that many bereaved people may find deeply upsetting.
- It takes no account of differing religious beliefs about the nature of death.

Although each of these criticisms is certainly valid, the journalist and agony aunt, Virginia Ironside, writing about her reactions to the death of her father, expresses her own objection in a very honest way and forthright way: 'my own instinctive feeling is that *you do not work through bereavement. It works through you*'[5] (author's italics).

This description, and Ironside's assertion that the *passivity* involved in bereavement is the most frightening aspect, probably strikes a chord with many bereaved people: 'the feeling that something terrible is being done to you – which it is'[5]

Individual responses to bereavement: continuing bonds

More recently, the idea of attempting to impose order on emotions, particularly notions of 'letting go' and 'recovery', has been challenged not just by academics but also by other bereaved people who, like Ironside, have chosen to share their experiences of grieving with others. What has gradually emerged is an understanding that bereaved people respond to the death of a loved one in a very *individual* way, and that there can be neither *rules* about grieving nor universal *models* of the process.

Consider the following account:

> I was in a new world, with a new language and new emotions. Perhaps he [the deceased] was resting in peace, but I was in utter turmoil. I was stunned and crazy. Not with grief, which, it turned out, was only a small part of the whole ghastly process, but with other shameful feelings of rage, greed, loathing, hatred for life – and with new, surprising interests in religion and the afterlife.[5]

The same writer talks of how her bereavement has left her, 18 months later, living in a land of 'grief, rage and confusion.' She wonders whether she is destined to live there forever, or whether bereavement is actually a journey and that she will eventually land in another port. Certainly this description of being totally adrift and beset with a whole range of unfamiliar, terrifying and continually changing emotions – not just grief – and with no end in sight, is very common. What seems particularly difficult for bereaved people to deal with is the sense of being on a rollercoaster of emotions and totally out of control, as well as a terrible suspicion that they have gone completely crazy. The way in which a welcome period of feeling more cheerful and optimistic can be just as suddenly followed by a return of the types of overwhelming feelings described above can be particularly distressing.

What is also apparent from personal accounts of bereavement is that, even in the midst of frightening and unfamiliar emotional turmoil, many people do not want to 'let go' of the past, but strive to maintain *continuing bonds* with the deceased person.[6] The bereaved individual gradually finds a way to incorporate the memory of the relationship with the loved one into his or her life while continuing to carry out necessary daily tasks and striving to build a new and different life in which the deceased is no longer present. In that sense, there is no danger that the dead person will ever be forgotten, but the maintenance of bonds may provide a way for grief to be accepted and the loss gradually assimilated. It is interesting that some people choose public expression of their continuing bond, while others find private ways to maintain their memories (*see* Box 13.4). Some may draw comfort from both.

Box 13.4 Some ways of maintaining continuing bonds

In public
Tending a grave on a regular basis
Planting a tree, rosebush or evergreen plant
Newspaper memorials on the anniversary of the death or the deceased's birthday
Regular donations to a charity in memory of the deceased

In private
Talking to the deceased's photograph
Privately asking the deceased's opinion on important matters and feeling that he or she has responded
Visiting the deceased's favourite place
Keeping a special memento of the deceased, such as a watch or piece of jewellery

---

Reflection Exercise 13.2

What were you taught about reactions to bereavement? How does this relate to your own or others' experiences of bereavement?

Ethnic minorities and bereavement

The UK is a multi-ethnic, multicultural society, and it is important for health and social care professionals to consider how members of other faith communities (e.g. Hindus, Sikhs, Muslims, Buddhists) understand death and experience bereavement. Despite the variety and complexity of different belief systems, there are several common factors.

• All of the major world religions teach that there is some kind of continuity or life after death, and their various mourning and bereavement rituals often reflect this.

- Different cultures or faiths acknowledge the need for the expression of emotion in bereavement, even though this may sometimes legitimately take the form of anger or aggression rather than tears.
- There is almost always practical acknowledgement that bereaved individuals or families need emotional support and comfort for varying periods of time, although this is reflected in different ways in different faiths.
- Some religions or cultures offer a final ceremony which signals the official end of the mourning period, although they may continue to mark the anniversary of the death in some way.

It is obviously important to be able to exhibit cultural sensitivity and understanding towards bereaved people of other faiths, and to appreciate that *personal grief* may be different to *culturally required mourning*. However, mere knowledge of the mourning and bereavement rituals of different faiths may not be sufficient. Members of a PHCT need to be able to recognise how the experience of living in a different society, with its own beliefs, expectations and practices, increased mobility and the gradual fragmentation of traditional family structures, may mean that the customs and rituals associated with mourning and bereavement in a particular faith community may change over a period of time. Scrutton[7] recommends checking with each individual concerning their personal beliefs and expectations about mourning and bereavement, rather than making assumptions based on stereotypical thinking and possible misinformation.

Reflection Exercise 13.3

What mourning and bereavement customs or rituals prevail in your culture or faith? Are these changing in any way? If so, why might this be?

Risk factors in bereavement

A considerable number of studies have been conducted, mainly in the USA, which have tried to establish whether there are any factors that are associated with increased health risk and other poor outcomes following bereavement. However, the available data need to be interpreted with some caution due to the following:

- the differing methodological approaches involved and their validity
- the lack of reliable measures of bereavement outcomes
- the different settings in which various studies have been conducted.

Bearing these difficulties in mind, it is possible to summarise briefly the current state of knowledge and to identify the factors which have been implicated in creating particularly adverse reactions in the bereaved, although more longitudinal studies would be required to assess any *long-term* health outcomes.

Box 13.5   Risk factors in bereavement (adapted from Sanders[8])

Mode of death	Sudden death, including suicide, murder, catastrophe and stigmatised death (e.g. from AIDS) may cause prolonged grief and trauma
Ambivalence and dependency	'Unfinished business' with the deceased, resulting in self-reproach and guilt, or intense fear of being left alone and being unable to cope
Parental bereavement	Mothers appear to grieve more deeply than fathers, perhaps on account of deeply ingrained bonding with the child; this causes enormous immediate disruption in the family, but any physical symptoms may not emerge for many years
Health before bereavement	If a person's health was poor before bereavement, it is likely that the stress of grief will exaggerate the condition, but there is more evidence for the effects on physical health than for those on mental health. Evidence to date derives primarily from clinical or anecdotal sources
Concurrent crises	Where bereavement is accompanied by other stressful losses (e.g. redundancy, financial problems, divorce, etc.)
Perceived lack of social support	May be particularly relevant to elderly people, especially if they are isolated, but immediate relatives are not always the best source of support
Age and gender	Studied mainly in the context of spousal bereavement — problems may be different at different ages. Widowers seem to thrive less well than widows
Reduced material resources	Particularly relevant to widows, whose socio-economic circumstances may change on the death of a spouse; also a risk factor for depression

---

It is likely that *personality* factors also play a part in how a bereaved person copes with the death of a loved one. The risk of a poor outcome may be reduced if a person is adaptable, resilient and optimistic about their ability to carry on. There is less evidence as to whether *religious belief* is helpful with regard to coping with loss although, as previously discussed, membership of a faith community may offer a source of support and a prescribed set of bereavement rituals.

Grief reactions

The risk factors identified above can be a useful guide for members of the PHCT who are faced with a bereaved patient, regardless of their age and circumstances. However, each bereavement is different, and the ways in which people cope with grief and the turmoil of emotions that may accompany it can also vary widely. Many bereaved people may be initially so overwhelmed by their loss that they begin to doubt whether they will ever function normally again. The expression of grief may take a variety of forms, and it is important that members of the primary care team are aware of the range of emotional and physical reactions that bereaved patients may suffer, and of the possible social impact of grief.

Table 13.1   The impact of grief (adapted from Scrutton[7])

Emotional reactions	Physical reactions	Social effects
Sorrow	Loss of appetite	Inability to cope with normal
Depression	(or over-eating)	social activities
Anxiety	Insomnia	Feeling overwhelmed
Anger	Exhaustion	A sense that life is futile
Regret	Inertia	Low self-esteem and
Guilt	Tension	self-interest
Despair	Restlessness	
Yearning	A variety of non-specific	
Fear	aches and pains	
Helplessness	Symptoms identified with	
Bitterness	those of the deceased's	
	final illness	

Obviously any symptoms which a recently bereaved patient reports need investigation, especially as there is some evidence that existing health problems can be exacerbated by the stress of bereavement and grief (*see* Box 13.5 above). Some people may also try to cope with their grief through over-reliance on alcohol or drugs, and this in turn may have various undesirable physical and/or emotional outcomes.

A special case: the death of a spouse or partner

In everyday practice, it is the death of a patient's *spouse or longstanding partner* that is most likely to be encountered. Whether sudden or anticipated, such a death can often cause the surviving partner to feel that the world is collapsing around them and that nothing makes sense any more. Survivors may often describe themselves as feeling as if they have had a limb amputated or as if their whole identity has been destroyed. In any case, it is important to remember the following points.

- The death of a spouse/partner has far-reaching social, economic and possibly health-related implications, some of which will inevitably impact upon the rest of the survivor's life, even if a new partnership is eventually formed.
- The ending of a committed relationship through death of one of the partners can be a heavy burden to bear at any age, and may pose unique emotional and practical problems at different points of the life course. However, it is ageist to assume that elderly people are accustomed to loss and do not need support in the same way as younger people. At the same time, it is patronising to assume that they cannot make decisions about their future and must be protected from grief.
- The potential difficulties faced by the surviving partner of a gay or lesbian relationship should not be underestimated, especially if the relatives had been unaware of the relationship or hostile to it in some way, so that the surviving partner is excluded from grief and mourning rituals.

The emotional, physical and social impact of grief may be heightened for a bereaved spouse/partner who may also be coping with the grief of children and other family members. In addition to the grief symptoms described above, surviving partners often experience a range of sensations that they are afraid to mention due to embarrassment or a fear that they might be going mad. Initially these might include the following:

- hallucinations of the deceased or a sense of his or her presence in the house
- complete loss of sex drive or, conversely, a heightened sense of desire which may provoke feelings of guilt and shame
- a sense of unreality accompanied by complete inertia and inability to make decisions.

Later on, the following might be experienced:

- an overwhelming sense of loneliness and isolation
- sheer exhaustion from the efforts involved in dealing with officialdom in the aftermath of the death.

Bereavement care in the community

In most cases it is the PHCT that is the immediate point of contact for a bereaved spouse/partner and his or her family, or indeed for any person who has endured the loss of a loved one. However, in recent years there has been a growth in the provision of professional support and counselling services for the bereaved, as well as expansion of the services offered by the hospice movement. When considering the type of additional support that a bereaved patient might need, it is useful to consider the whole range of possible sources of assistance.

- *Relatives, friends, neighbours and/or work colleagues.* Most people have a supportive network whose members will rally round during the early stages of bereavement, and who can offer appropriate comfort, support and practical help. However, as time goes by, many bereaved people often find that it is assumed that they have 'recovered' or 'got over it'. As they appear to be rebuilding their lives, other family members and friends may gradually withdraw their support, unaware that bereaved people often need to talk about their loss and to have their pain acknowledged long after they appear to have returned to some sort of normality. Some people also find that former friends avoid them or that work colleagues find it difficult to mention the bereavement. Others, particularly widows, may sometimes be distressed by the well-meaning but tactless comments of friends and acquaintances.

- *Counselling.* Although it is sometimes available within primary care, this is now usually provided by trained volunteers supported by professionals through local Bereavement Care Services – often under the auspices of CRUSE, the largest voluntary bereavement counselling organisation in the UK. Although it should never be assumed that a bereaved person automatically needs counselling, many people find this helpful for a short period, especially as it provides the opportunity to talk freely about feelings outside the confines of the immediate family. Bereavement counselling has been influenced by a variety of disciplines in recent years, but mainly focuses on helping bereaved individuals to explore, express and understand their emotions so that they can gradually come to terms with their loss.

- *Telephone helplines.* There is now a wide range of organisations that offer confidential telephone helplines for bereaved people, staffed by trained volunteers who have suffered a particular type of bereavement themselves. These range from the Child Death Helpline for anyone affected by the death of a child, no matter how long ago, to the Blue Cross Pet Bereavement Support Service, which provides support and compassion for people mourning the loss of a companion animal. Callers to such helplines are given the opportunity to express their feelings and concerns and to receive non-judgemental acceptance and reassurance from someone who can empathise from personal experience.

- *Self-help groups.* These are groups in which bereaved people organise support and perhaps a programme of social activities for other bereaved individuals, sometimes with the support of professionals but often on the initiative of one particular person. The National Association of Widows provides an umbrella for some self-help groups, and some funeral services now offer these types of opportunities as part of their continuing commitment to bereaved people, whether or not their services were originally used.

- *The Internet.* This is also increasingly a unique source of support for those who have suffered a loss. It is now possible to communicate electronically with other bereaved people without having to reveal one's identity (e.g. through Grief-Chat and WidowNet). Although not everyone would find this an acceptable outlet for the expression of grief, it may increasingly come to provide an invaluable source of support for those who would find it difficult to articulate their needs or ask for help from more conventional sources.

Reflection Exercise 13.4

If you have suffered a bereavement, who or what was your major source of support? Did your needs for support change over time?

Implications of bereavement for the PHCT

Any death affects a whole range of people for a long time, whatever their relationship to the deceased. A primary care practice might therefore wish to review its strategies to plan for addressing the needs of bereaved patients in a supportive and caring manner over a lengthy period of time.

Managing bereavement in primary care

In the immediate aftermath of a death
- Pay a home visit to offer condolences immediately after a death. This provides:
  (i) an acknowledgement of the loss, and reassurance that there is a source of support
  (ii) an opportunity for family members to discuss the circumstances of the death and/or clarify any clinical details and receive reassurance about emotional reactions if necessary and/or ask for information about legal/cremation procedures.
- Be aware of any religious or cultural requirements (discussed above).
- Consider the possible need for sedation (now rarely prescribed unless the circumstances of the death were particularly sudden and distressing), and for sick leave for employed family members if appropriate.
- Make a record in the notes of immediate family members. This may be important at future consultations.
- Arrange another visit to take place in a few weeks' time, but emphasise that a member of the PHCT can be available at any time before that if necessary.

After 2 to 3 weeks
- Visit the family again. If a spouse/partner is now alone, it *may* be helpful to suggest sources of practical and/or emotional support (see above). Suggest tactfully that no major decisions (e.g. on moving house/entering residential care) should be made for at least a year, but remember that bereaved people do not always respond rationally to ideas that were meant to be helpful.
- Listen to any concerns of different family members in private if possible.
- Offer advice on general health, including that of any children, if this is deemed necessary.
- Make an appointment for a member of the team to visit again at a convenient time.

After 6 weeks

- Another member of the team may wish to visit to give reassurance about grief reactions and concerns about any children or young people.
- Be prepared to answer questions or engage in frank discussion of issues which may be troubling the bereaved. The sense of being on an emotional roller-coaster often begins to emerge at this time.
- If a bereaved individual acted as the deceased's carer, he or she may feel particularly isolated if support from health and/or social care services has abruptly ceased. It may help if support services keep in touch, even if only by telephone, for as long as is practically possible.
- Encourage and promote self-care, healthy eating and physical exercise.
- Encourage the fostering of supportive relationships with others.
- Encourage ways of maintaining bonds with the deceased (*see* Box 13.4 above), but only if this is mentioned by family members.
- Watch out for any signs of deep depression, self-neglect and self-harm or the emergence of suicidal thoughts, especially in bereaved spouses/partners and older people.

Over the first 2 years

- Be aware of risk factors (*see* Box 13.5 above) if a bereaved patient presents with symptoms of ill health at any time.
- Arrange for a member of the team to telephone or visit briefly on the anniversary of the death. Other difficult times are often other personal anniversaries, birthdays and holiday times, especially the first Christmas after the bereavement. Check that the bereaved person will not be alone at holiday times (unless they wish it – some do prefer to spend the time quietly reminiscing).
- Check unobtrusively whether a bereaved spouse/partner has resumed or is rebuilding a social life. Some people may need considerable help in making new contacts and friends, especially bereaved spouses/partners who may have been used to doing everything as a couple (*see* page 186 for sources of assistance).·
- At future routine consultations, enquire after the well-being of family members. Bereaved people need to know that their grief and changed circumstances have not been forgotten. Never assume that they have 'got over it,' however cheerful they may seem to be.

Final remarks

Any kind of loss can be very distressing and have repercussions that may impinge on an individual's life in a variety of ways for a lengthy period of time. However, the death of a loved one is probably the most devastating of human experiences – yet it is something that everyone must experience sooner or later. With sensitive and timely support, many people emerge from the experience of bereavement with a new sense of pride and self-confidence in their ability to cope with adversity. In order to provide that support, members of the PHCT need to be comfortable with their own mortality and with the emotions that exposure to dying and death can raise. In particular, they need to consider the following:

- their own spiritual beliefs about life and death
- where to find support if it is needed
- how to use that support as an important part of everyday professional practice.

References

1 Hockey J, Katz J and Small N (2001) *Grief, Mourning and Death Ritual*. Open University Press, Buckingham.
2 Parkes CM (1986) *Bereavement: studies of grief in adult life*. Penguin Books, Harmondsworth.
3 Kübler-Ross E (1969) *On Death and Dying*. Macmillan, New York.
4 Worden JW (1982) *Grief Counselling and Grief Therapy: a handbook for the mental health practitioner*. Springer, New York.
5 Ironside V (1996) *'You'll Get Over It'. The rage of bereavement*. Penguin Books, Harmondsworth.
6 Klass D, Silverman PR and Nickman SL (1996) *Continuing Bonds: new understandings of grief*. Taylor & Francis, Washington, DC.
7 Scrutton S (1995) *Bereavement and Grief. Supporting older people through loss*. Edward Arnold, London.
8 Sanders CM (1993) Risk factors in bereavement outcome. In: MS Stroebe, W Stroebe and RO Hansson (eds) *Handbook of Bereavement. Theory, research and intervention*. Cambridge University Press, Cambridge.

Useful website

www.bbc.co.uk/education/archive/grave/index.html: BBC website with information on what to do when someone dies, and on coping with bereavement.

CHAPTER 14

Drawing up and applying a personal development plan (PDP) in palliative care

Rodger Charlton

Background

Continuing professional development (CPD) is a new acronym where definitions and potential applications abound. CPD is a process built on the philosophy of lifelong learning (LLL), and it needs to be differentiated from continuing medical education (CME) as it is referred to by the medical Royal Colleges. This is because CPD involves more than attending teaching sessions, as it also entails personal and professional development by regular formative appraisal identifying learning needs, reflective practice, the gaining of new knowledge and skills, and application of the philosophy of LLL.

CPD and general practitioners

CPD for GPs currently involves a voluntary system of attending 30 hours of accredited courses or learning activity annually, which was introduced in 1990 with the 'New Contract'. In order for GPs to earn a proportion of their income, they had to attend 30 hours of approved postgraduate education, which was referred to as the postgraduate education allowance (PGEA).

The Department of Health, following the Chief Medical Officer's report on CPD in 1998, has suggested a move from the traditional CME for GPs leading to the PGEA. This is by a transition to the accreditation of personal learning plans (PLPs), also more correctly referred to as personal development plans (PDPs), through local GP tutors.

At the present time there are five categories of GPs in relation to the existing PGEA system:

1 those who have been gaining accreditation of their PLPs for several years to substitute for the PGEA
2 doctors who have written and submitted approved PDPs this year
3 doctors who have written but not submitted approved PDPs this year

4   doctors who will remain with the old 'PGEA system' until the contractual requirements change

5   the small minority who are not involved in the 'PGEA system' of activity.

The existing PGEA system and personal learning plans

Until now, the 'PGEA system' has provided a 'quick fix' to what should be a more structured long-term view of our CPD. Furthermore, it has not necessarily been tailored to meet GPs' learning needs or relevant to their practice. This PGEA learning activity has often been haphazard rather than structured, and now the recommendation is the construction of personal learning plans. PLPs have the potential to provide a more structured long-term view of our CPD. Therefore qualifications such as medical degrees, postgraduate training and the MRCGP diploma should not be seen as end points, but rather as the initiation of lifelong learning. CPD should involve the updating of knowledge and the gaining new skills.

It could be said that attendance at PGEA meetings or lectures is based on a ritual, a free lunch and inadequate time to devote to CPD. The educational content is based on clinical interests or what could be described as 'comfy niches', rather than on learning needs in a particular aspect of clinical practice. The traditional didactic methods of a medical lecture could be criticised, as they can encourage passive as opposed to active learning.

The shift in focus needs to be towards personal and professional development needs and a philosophy of adult learning which is moving away from the traditional pedagogical model and didactic teaching styles, and thus a shift of responsibility for learning from teacher to adult learner using innovative methods of learning such as reflection and portfolio development. In addition, academic knowledge only becomes professional knowledge when it is applied practically in the clinical context.

The very nature of general practice, whether practised solo or in groups, can lead to professional isolation. There is a need to be self-reliant, self-critical and self-directed in GPs' professional development and learning, and there is encouragement of GPs to take responsibility for their own learning. CPD is concerned with this through the constant updating of professional knowledge throughout an individual's working life, requiring self-direction, self-management and a responsiveness to the development opportunities that are offered by work experience.

CPD in nursing

The UK Central Council for Nursing, Midwifery and Health Visiting (UKCC) stipulates that nurses have to update their professional skills regularly in order to stay on the register. The UKCC's post-registration education and practice (PREP) requirements involve nurses undertaking the equivalent of a minimum of 35 hours of continuing professional development over a period of three years. Details of this should be kept in a personal professional portfolio (e.g. activities such as study days, unstructured learning, work experience and current projects).

The UKCC's five recommended study areas are as follows:

- reducing risk
- care enhancement
- patient, client and colleague support
- practice development
- education development.

Like general practice, the nursing profession has its own terminology. Continuing education points (CEPs) are awarded by the Royal College of Nursing (RCN) for activity that has been accredited by the RCN Institute. They are a clear indication that work has been recognised as being of high quality. CEPs also represent a period of study time – two CEPs represent one hour of RCN-accredited CPD activity. Further details are available from the RCN website (www.rcn.org.uk). It should be noted that the UKCC register is soon to become the Nursing and Midwifery Council (NMC).

CPD and healthcare professionals

CPD schemes are not study programmes or ways to encourage people to attend a lot of courses. They are about enabling healthcare professionals to reflect on their own personal and professional development needs, their workplace development needs and how those needs can be met. The objectives of CPD should be linked to an increase in knowledge and skills with regard to caring for patients. An overall goal should be to improve the capabilities of the whole team, so in addition to a PDP an individual practitioner's educational objectives should be part of a practice professional development plan (PPDP).

Many professions now run CPD schemes, and different professions use different names for CPD. PDPs appear to have evolved from industry and the teaching profession. The methods that are employed by healthcare professionals and their professional bodies to facilitate CPD through PDPs have therefore been imported from other professions.

How does one draw up a PDP?

Many different pro formas exist for these plans, and ideally they should also form part of or relate to the practice professional development plan. In each situation it is important that individual practitioners (e.g. GPs) identify their own learning needs and, where appropriate, relate them to the learning needs of the associated primary healthcare teams (PHCTs). It may be helpful to sit down with a colleague and peer who is trained in this area (e.g. the local postgraduate centre tutor or the local primary care group/trust (PCG/T) tutor) in order to appraise a practitioner's knowledge and skills in an area such as palliative care. It is important to define what is meant by appraisal, as perceptions and interpretations differ widely. Appraisal, if correctly applied, is not an assessment, but rather a method of valuing quality. Appraisal should be formative rather than summative. It should be aimed at development, not assessment – otherwise it is not an appraisal but a management tool.

When a GP or practitioner meets with the person conducting such an educational appraisal, a potential PDP should be discussed on the basis of perceived learning needs, and an action plan relating to development in the future should be considered and mutually agreed.

Pro forma for PDP

There are several different pro formas or templates available. The simpler they are, the easier they are to complete and use. It is helpful when writing a PDP to focus on the following areas:

- identification of learning needs
- educational objectives
- learning strategy or strategies to meet needs
- how objectives relate to the PPDP
- resources required
- estimated time-scale
- expected outcomes and evidence or portfolio of objectives being met, and thus CPD
- importance for PHCT and dissemination.

Worked example in palliative care

When considering a PDP for yourself, of which palliative care may form a part or a whole, the following factors need to be considered.

- Is the duration of your plan one year or five years?
- Have you talked to, for example, the local GP tutor?
- Have you discussed with the tutor whether your plan (PDP) can be accredited to receive the postgraduate education allowance (PGEA)?
- Will other members of the PHCT be involved in your PDP?
- Will your plan relate to patient care?
- If your PDP has been accredited for CPD (PGEA for GPs), have you posted it together with the necessary fee to your regional director of postgraduate education in general practice (previously known as your regional adviser in general practice)?

Identification of learning needs

The most important part of your PDP is the identification of your learning needs. This can be done in conjunction with other members of the PHCT and could, for example, be discussed at a practice meeting. You could raise areas in which you perceive you have learning needs and ask if these are the same for other members of the PHCT, or whether other members of the team have skills in these areas.

In addition, you should consider as a team the possible implications and also the potential benefits for patient care, and how the PDP could feed into that care.

The drawing up of a PDP can be summarised as follows.

- Identify learning needs.
- Discuss these with other members of the PHCT at a practice meeting.
- Consider the implications for patient care.
- Discuss the PDP with, for example, the GP tutor.

Palliative care as an example of a PDP

Palliative care is a philosophy of care that is applicable to many disease conditions in addition to cancer. It has potential application to any progressive life-threatening disease in which curative (active) therapy is no longer possible and therapy is now aimed at palliation. It is the transition from curative to palliative therapy that is fraught with dilemmas for the patient, informal carers and professional carers and leads to the focus on the philosophy of palliative care.

Examples of such diseases include the following:

- cancer-related disease
- chronic obstructive pulmonary disease (COPD)
- multiple sclerosis (MS)
- motor neurone disease (MND)
- acquired immunodeficiency syndrome (AIDS)
- Alzheimer's-type dementia
- rare neurological conditions, such as variant Creutzfeldt–Jakob disease (vCJD).

The term 'palliative medicine' rather than 'care' is misleading in that it may give the impression of a doctor-led movement with an emphasis on symptom control. There is now a shifting paradigm from medicalisation to total care or 'supportive care'. Of necessity this will involve other members of the healthcare team, so that 'total care' is provided with an equal emphasis on nursing, emotional, social, psychological and spiritual needs as well as the physical needs. This ensures that the patient has the best possible quality of life until they die, and provides support for their family and carers.

Identifying learning needs in palliative care

This book discusses important areas of palliative care in depth, and some readers will already have identified some chapters as learning needs. Some may say that a large proportion of primary care is palliative care – hence the title of the book:

Primary Palliative Care. However, that does not make one an expert, and it is important to be aware of deficiencies in knowledge and skills in palliative care.

Identifying learning needs in a specific area of palliative care

When constructing a PDP, there is likely to be more than one topic or area covered by the PDP, and there may well be a link to local and national needs in relation to clinical governance and the National Service Frameworks (NSFs) (e.g. the NSF for Diabetes). Thus when considering a topic as wide-ranging as palliative care, it might be worth asking how this large and broad topic relates to another large and broad topic (e.g. primary diabetes care).

Learning needs in the overlap between palliative care and diabetes

Diabetes is a disease condition that should be treated actively, bearing in mind the results of the UK Prospective Diabetes Study (UKPDS) in 1998 and the need to achieve tight glycaemic and blood pressure control. However, on occasions complications of diabetes occur, and treatment is then aimed at palliation if cure is no longer possible (e.g. in cases of chronic painful neuropathy).

Contemplating learning needs

Is there something new or an area that you have not previously considered in relation to the topics of palliative care and diabetes that has arisen from your clinical practice?

Identifying learning needs

When thinking about my own learning needs and my own clinical practice, I identified three areas that relate to palliative care and diabetes. This led to three questions where I needed to find out more information that has relevance to my own practice and its PPDP, and so to the practice team. This will now be discussed in depth to illustrate how a PDP might be written, using palliative care and its overlap with diabetes as a worked example. When considering a learning plan in relation to diabetes and how this relates to palliative care, the following three questions could be asked.

1   Patients with type II diabetes have a progressive disease with increasing failure of insulin production, increasing insulin resistance and its associated sequelae. Is there a point at which diabetes goes beyond active treatment and a patient with diabetes requires the principles of palliation (e.g. for intractable pain from end-stage neuropathy or renal failure or heart failure)? At what point is palliation more important than the rigours of tight glycaemic control advocated traditionally and confirmed by the UKPDS study? These are perhaps dilemmas that healthcare professionals do not consider, as it may not be contemplated that a patient may enter a 'terminal' phase as a result of their diabetes, and that consequently palliation might be the best option for providing optimum quality of life. The issue of whether there are situations for patients with diabetes where palliation has a role must be discussed with the active involvement of the patient and their carers. The founder of the modern hospice movement, Dame Cicely Saunders, suggests that palliative treatment should enable a person to 'live until they die'. This is relevant, as all people with diabetes have the potential to develop complications which are irreversible and may in themselves threaten life.

2   A certain proportion of patients with diabetes develop cancer and eventually may start to receive palliative care. Anecdotally I have the impression that the rigours of tight glycaemic control are neglected when a person with diabetes receives palliative care. Yet if palliative care is aimed at maintaining quality of life, perhaps the feeling of well-being may be enhanced by avoiding hyperglycaemia and associated symptoms such as tiredness.

3   Certain cancers (e.g. carcinoma of the pancreas) and certain therapies used in palliative care (e.g. steroids) can lead to altered glycaemic control and thus to diabetes. How should people in palliative care scenarios such as these be managed in relation to glycaemic control? Again, should the rigours of tight glycaemic control be applied?

When identifying your learning needs, it is important not to choose such a large and broad topic as palliative care or diabetes, as there will not be adequate time to address such a large subject, particularly within one year, as in this worked example. Hence the rationale for looking at an aspect of care in a field where you believe you have little knowledge or skills, and so there is potential for improved patient care.

Implementing your PDP

Having identified the learning needs that relate to you as an individual practitioner, the PHCT with whom you work and thus the PPDP, you should:

- discuss and reflect on them with a clinical tutor
- decide on a learning strategy or strategies
- state your learning objectives
- consider a realistic time-scale
- draw up an action plan in the form of a PDP
- define outcomes and thus the achievement of objectives.

PDP action plan based on identified needs of patients with diabetes and palliative care

The worked example on page 199 is presented as a pro forma. There are many PDP pro formas available, but no recommended format as yet. The learning strategies employed indicate methods that suit me personally, but may not suit other practitioners. PDPs should be individual to each practitioner, so there may be aspects with which the reader does not concur. Other strategies may include Internet computer searches, reading of the literature, spending time with a specialist, going on a course or attending a didactic lecture. The success of a PDP can be measured in terms of knowledge acquired and new skills gained and thus CPD, and therefore their potential application to improving patient care and application in the practice, locally and perhaps also nationally. It is these aspects of learning that will enable a practitioner to measure whether their objectives have been achieved. Finally, when writing a PDP, bear in mind the workload of a busy clinician and consider realistic time-scales.

Time allocation and summary of PGEA requirements

- Painful neuropathy – 4 hours Disease Management, 5 hours Health Promotion, 3 hours Service Management.
- Cancer patients with diabetes – 3 hours Disease Management, 5 hours Health Promotion, 4 hours Service Management.
- Induced diabetes in cancer patients – 3 hours Disease Management, 3 hours Service Management.

Total: 10 hours Disease Management, 10 hours Health Promotion and 10 hours Service Management.
Overall: 30 hours of learning to claim the PGEA through an accredited PDP.

Conclusion

There is no standard method for producing a PDP, and different regions employ different pro formas. Your local GP tutor will be able to advise you as to whether a plan such as this can be accredited. This is a worked example to illustrate learning needs in the overlapping area of palliative care and diabetes. It is not my own personal PDP, and this example has not been accredited. It has been written to illustrate the process and to highlight issues relating to palliative care and diabetes, an area on which little has been written. This example fits nicely into a learning cycle, and following its implementation it may be applied where appropriate to clinical practice and the PPDP, and finally reflected upon, which may help to identify further learning needs.

Personal development plan (PDP)

Learning needs/ gaps identified	Learning objectives – desired achievements	Learning methods	Application to team PPDP and PCG/PCT	Resources required	Timetable/time-scales	Measured success – evidence of achieving objective and CPD	Importance for patient care – making findings known (dissemination)
Painful neuropathy in patients with diabetes	• To identify patients – creation of a register • To gain knowledge of the subject • Audit of care of patients on register and development of scale of care provided	• Use of computers and involvement of PHCT members • Literature search • Conducting an audit • Clinical session with a specialist	• Awareness of painful neuropathy • Education in the area • Taking part in an audit	• Time • Diabetes register • Practice meeting to explain project • Assistance with audit and computer • Medical library	12 hours over 12 months	• Disease register • Collection of literature summarised • The audit data	• Reducing symptoms in this group • Discussion of findings at practice meeting • Report to go to clinical governance lead in PCG/PCT
Cancer patients with diabetes – their palliative care needs as a result of diabetes and cancer	• Identification of patients in the practice now and in the past • Creation of records/ charts/registers of patients with cancer who require palliative care, in particular those with diabetes • Creation of record of those diabetes patients who have died of cancer • Creation of a death register	• Use of computers and involvement of PHCT members • Audit of diabetes patients with diabetes and also those who have died as a result of diabetes-related complications	• Increased computer skills • Education and awareness in this area • Taking part in an audit	• Time • Good records • Recall of records from PCG/PCT and computer records • Assistance with audit and computer • Medical library	12 hours over 12 months	• Creation of record of patients • Audit of this area to ascertain level of diabetes care in relation to palliation • Death register	• Reducing symptoms in this group • Discussion of findings at practice meeting • Report to go to clinical governance lead in PCG/PCT • Creation of a death register which may have other applications (e.g. in bereavement)
Induced diabetes in cancer patients	• The use of steroids in palliative care • To learn more about diabetes as a result of pancreatic cancer	• Clinical session with a palliative medicine specialist • Literature searches	• Awareness of the problem and use of steroids in palliative care	• Time • Friendly palliative medicine consultant!	6 hours over 12 months	• Details of session/ sessions with palliative medicine consultant • Collection of literature summarised	• Discussion of findings at practice meeting • Report to go to clinical governance lead in PCG/PCT • Application to patient care in the future

Doctor's name: Dr Rodger Charlton, The Surgery, Hampton-in-Arden, Solihull.

Further reading

- Benbow SJ, Cossins L and MacFarlane IA (1999) Painful diabetic neuropathy. *Diabetic Med.* **16**: 632–44.
- Bornman PC and Beckingham IJ (2001) ABC of diseases of liver, pancreas and biliary system: pancreatic tumours. *BMJ.* **322**: 721–3.
- Boyd K (1993) Diabetes mellitus in hospice patients: some guidelines. *Palliative Med.* **7**: 163–4.
- Charlton R (2001) Continuing professional development (CPD) and training. *BMJ.* **323 (Career Focus 18 August)**: S2–3.
- de Grauw WJ, van de Lisdonk EH, van Gerwen WH, van den Hoogen HJ and van Weel C (2001) Insulin therapy in poorly controlled type 2 diabetic patients: does it affect quality of life? *Br J Gen Pract.* **51**: 527–32.
- Dunning T (1996) Corticosteroid medications and diabetes mellitus. *Pract Diabetes Int.* **13**: 186–8.
- Kessler I (1971) Cancer and diabetes mellitus: a review of the literature. *J Chron Dis.* **23**: 579–600.
- Kitzes JA (2000) Diabetes mellitus: palliative care strategies. *Ind Health Serv Provider.* **January**: 2–4.
- Kovner V (1998) Management of diabetes in advanced cancer: urine sugar tests. *J Pain Symptom Manage.* **15**: 147–8.
- Poulson J (1997) The management of diabetes in patients with advanced cancer. *J Pain Symptom Manage.* **13**: 339–46.
- Rughani A (2001) *The GP's Guide to Personal Development Plans* (2e). Radcliffe Medical Press, Oxford.

CHAPTER 15

Teamwork and education through significant event audit (SEA) and practice professional development plans (PPDPs)

John Wilmot and Karen Mills

Importance of teamworking

Consider the case of two men in their sixties with malignant disease. One of them, a married, retired professional, has a slowly progressive condition and is active until the last few weeks of his life. After initial diagnosis he receives his hospital care from the oncology team, while he sees his general practitioner and district nurse regularly. Eventually he is admitted to the oncology unit because of worsening symptoms, and he dies there. Two health teams (oncology and primary care) therefore look after him. The second patient is an unemployed divorced factory worker who lives alone. As well as lung cancer he has ischaemic heart disease. He is admitted to hospital often with chest pain and breathlessness. These symptoms are sometimes attributed to either of his two major conditions, and anxiety is often thought to play a major part in them. Thus many teams (palliative care, cardiology, medical and of course primary care) are involved in the care of the second patient.

It can be seen that teams ('small groups of people with a common goal or task') play an important part in palliative care. Although teams are important, they do not always function efficiently or harmoniously. Similarly, the teams in different places often do not communicate well or work in the desirable 'seamless' fashion.

Problems with teams

Doctors, nurses and administrative staff work together, representing the basic unit that provides healthcare. Family doctors in the UK commonly work in groups of between four and six, and the associated primary healthcare team (PHCT) will number between 20 and 30. Researchers from differing backgrounds have identified various problems in PHCTs, including poor communication, ignorance of one another's skills and roles, and a lack of clear or shared goals.[1]

Is it in fact appropriate to talk about the primary healthcare *team*? It may be more sensible to think of this grouping as a small organisation composed of separate although overlapping teams. Increasingly, nurses working in the community in the UK will work in 'integrated nursing teams' that seek to blur some traditional boundaries (e.g. between district nurses and health visitors).[2]

What can help PHCTs to avoid the above problems?

- *Climate and values* – an atmosphere of respect for members can be fostered. Opportunities can be taken for members to describe their skills and roles.
- Clear *communication channels* are helpful. These can include telephone, fax and computers, but face-to-face contact remains paramount.
- At *regular meetings* information can be shared and a group identity can be developed.
- *Joint learning* can be fostered – this is described in more detail below.
- *Social events* outside working hours can improve the team climate.

Education and the PHCT

> CPD is a process of lifelong learning for individuals and teams which enables them to develop personally and professionally, and to improve care for patients.[6]

Innovative educational approaches, including portfolios, personal learning plans and practice professional development plans, are becoming more familiar in primary care. A seminal report in 1998 by Kenneth Calman, Chief Medical Officer for England, encouraged such more novel methods.[3] He led a working group which advocated a new, broader approach to continuous professional development. The group's findings were much influenced by literature reviews which showed that passive methods such as lectures had little effect in improving patient care.[4] However, interactive methods are more effective.

Traditional continuing medical education (CME) has also concentrated almost exclusively on the updating of clinical knowledge. Today this may not be adequate, given current rapid changes in both technology and public expectations. Health professionals need to develop their abilities in communication, teamworking and information technology. These, like any other skills, are best learned through practice and feedback, often when working in small groups.

Adults are often seen as preferring particular learning approaches (more 'hands on' or interactive) that are geared towards solving the problems which they encounter in their daily lives. As 'self-directed' learners, adults often prefer to gain new knowledge and skills close to their workplaces, also learning together with their colleagues.[5] The Government sees lifelong learning for health workers as one of the chief routes to improving quality in the National Health Service.[6]

The assessment of educational needs

Health professionals can link their learning to problems experienced with patients, especially when these indicate educational needs. Richard Eve, a general practitioner tutor in Somerset, has described 'PUNs' and 'DENs'[©] that can be used in this way. One example would be a doctor visiting a terminally ill patient who is receiving opiate analgesia by continuous subcutaneous infusion. The syringe driver does not seem to be working, so the patient has troublesome pain. Unfortunately, the doctor lacks the knowledge to solve this problem directly. There will be both a patient's unmet need (PUN) in the form of unrelieved symptoms, and the doctor's educational need (DEN) to learn the basic skills of adjusting a syringe driver.[7]

Such methods are based on individual reflection on daily events. Feedback from colleagues can also help to develop an appreciation of educational needs (e.g. when questions are asked over a cup of coffee). Appraisal interviews or an ongoing relationship with a mentor are more structured methods for providing feedback to individuals. Until recently, appraisals have had very patchy application within the National Health Service, but the Government is now committed to introducing annual appraisal for all doctors, including general practitioners. Many nurses in the community (those employed by NHS trusts) undergo regular appraisal, and they also meet in groups for 'clinical supervision' as a form of co-mentoring.

Health needs assessment

The day-to-day learning of health professionals can and should be linked to the needs of patients, as described above. Likewise, overall planning for the education and development of the health team can be based on the health needs of the whole community. This may require the techniques of formal health needs assessment. Overall health service priorities, in the form of National Service Frameworks (NSFs) and local Health Improvement Plans (HImPs), should also inform the practice professional development plan (PPDP).

Significant event auditing (SEA)

Jane Smith was 45 years of age and had undergone surgery for breast cancer one year ago. During the following months she suffered increasingly severe low back pain. After several weeks she had an MRI scan which showed metastases in several lumbar vertebrae. One Thursday in August she requested a visit because of leg weakness. Her usual general practitioner visited her and observed that she could walk a few steps, although she was limping. He noted weak quadriceps, and considered that disuse atrophy was the cause of her problems. On the following Saturday another partner in the practice was called as Jane was having difficulty passing urine. He arranged for a district nurse to catheterise her, as she seemed to be developing urinary retention. The second doctor wondered about a referral to the oncologists, and decided that this should be put in hand after the weekend. When he telephoned the radiotherapy department on Monday, he was surprised how promptly Jane was admitted to hospital. Unfortunately, her spinal cord compression did not resolve with high-dose spinal radiotherapy, and she returned home in a paraplegic state.

Soon afterwards the practice held a significant event audit meeting. The doctors and nurses concerned were sad about the events that had affected Jane, and wondered whether they should have acted differently. The Macmillan nurse who was attached to the practice explained to the team about spinal cord compression, and how it affected 20% of patients with spinal metastases. A common sequence of events was for pain to be followed in turn by weakness, sensory loss, and disturbances of bowel and bladder function. She pointed out that consultant oncologists were on call each weekend expressly in order to deal with this problem.

Comment

Such a case would arouse strong feelings among those involved in this woman's healthcare. They would ask questions such as 'Did I do enough?', 'Was her treatment correct?' and 'Did we do the right things during that busy weekend on call?'.

Cases like the one described above receive attention from many primary care teams in significant event auditing. This is a case-based discussion method which enables team members to reflect on and learn from events which are emotionally disturbing, or which are related to the quality of the care that they provide.[8]

The principles of significant event auditing are therefore simple. A team that decides to use this method must first decide on events which it might consider, circulate recording sheets, and then hold meetings, perhaps monthly or bi-monthly. Different partners, the practice manager or other team members, depending on the skills that they possess, may facilitate the meetings. It is important to aim for a warm, supportive atmosphere, emphasising group learning and the improvement of care. Teamworking can benefit in a very direct way, while talking through disturbing events in this safe environment may ease work-related stress. As can be seen from the above case, the care of whole groups of patients may be improved in this way.[8-10]

Outline agenda for significant event meeting

- Acute/immediate care.
- Possibilities for prevention.
- Plan of action and follow-up.
- Implications for the team, other bodies/organisations or the community.

Table 15.1   Examples of events that could form the subject of significant event auditing

Clinical events	Organisational events
Deaths (expected or unexpected)	Patient complaint
Admission with asthma or diabetic ketosis	Home visit not made
Myocardial infarction or stroke	Failure to refer when agreed
Miscarriage	Lack of appointments

Experiences of cancer care using significant event audit

A total of 15 practices in Warwickshire used significant event audit (SEA) in a study of experiences of cancer care. The views of healthcare staff were combined with patients' views through semi-structured interviews performed by local Community Health Councils.

Study outline

In total, 15 practices (19% of 78 practices in the county) took part in the study. Various practice personnel attended a half-day training session to introduce them to the ideas and techniques of SEA. Each practice was asked to identify eight surviving patients, diagnosed within two years, with breast, lung, colorectal or prostate cancer. They were then asked to review, with all involved staff, the care of two patients at each of a series of SEA meetings over a period of one year.

The practices recorded the results of each meeting on a standard report form. They also completed a summary sheet to identify positive aspects, areas that needed improvement, and recommendations for acute care, possible prevention and follow-up, as well as wider implications for the team, other agencies and the community.

Findings

The practices utilised the significant event audit summary sheets to varying degrees, but some common themes could be identified from the aggregated data.

Instances were noted of both good practice and aspects needing improvement in the following areas:

- communication from hospital to GP about progress, planned treatments, and information given to the patient.
- communication between the PHCT and the patient and their family.

Recommendations included the following:

- a patient-held co-operation card to improve communication between all those involved in patient care
- increased use of fax facilities to speed up communication from consultant to PHCT.

Conclusions

The use of a structured significant event audit form proved successful in eliciting views from practices. Three out of the 15 practices taking part (20%) did not manage to complete any significant event audit forms. The practices themselves attributed this to difficulty in organising the necessary meetings. In these cases the practices may not have been ready to meet as a team to critically appraise the quality of care. It became apparent that using the SEA approach required a culture of trust and openness, to which these practices were not accustomed. More extended help from an external facilitator might help these practices to overcome such obstacles, and even to improve teamworking more generally. Additional support might also be needed to improve the process of SEA.[10]

Other learning methods

We all learn every day by reflecting on the patients we see, by talking about puzzling or unfamiliar aspects with colleagues, and by reading. In addition to these everyday activities, some educational methods are outlined below, with particular reference to those that can be applied in the practice setting.

In-practice education

Experts in particular fields (hospital consultants or others) could give presentations. They could be invited to discuss issues that are found troublesome by practitioners, rather than the latest scientific advances.[11] The smaller numbers and more informal setting should permit a much higher degree of interaction.

Practical skills

Sessions based on the demonstration and rehearsal of practical clinical skills (e.g. joint injections, cardiopulmonary resuscitation) may be more feasible in practices than elsewhere.

Communication

Workshops can be conducted for members of the primary healthcare team to help them to improve their communication skills. Video-recording equipment is now widely available (e.g. from postgraduate centres), and it may be useful to seek the services of a tutor or facilitator.

Audit and quality improvement

The team can discuss treatment goals in order to set audit standards, and then use the audit results to plan care changes. Significant event audit uses single cases or events in multidisciplinary meetings. Team members can consider organisation, communication and risk management. Small working groups within the larger team can apply continuous quality improvement methods. These will require them to study the processes involved in the care of patients, to reflect on their findings, and then to implement change.[12]

Formulating a PPDP: worked example

Practice professional development plans (PPDPs) are an innovation that was introduced following the publication of the Chief Medical Officer's report referred to above. Each primary care team would be expected to develop such a plan, agreed with a GP tutor or someone similar, each year. The PPDP could include practice-based and other novel forms of learning, and measures of learning needs and outcomes should also be included. Part of the aim of the Chief Medical Officer's report was to integrate the quality development of practices with their continuing education. Thus each plan should reflect service development plans for the practice, the locality and more widely. Ideally, it should be linked with the practice annual report, and should take into account both local and national priorities. It should be focused on long-term or at least medium-term development of the primary care team, its members and the services offered to patients.

For each topic that is included in a PPDP, there will be questions to be answered such as the following.

- *How was the topic identified*? Was this a result of team discussion, analysis of PACT or other data, a patient complaint, or advice from the health authority, patient advisory group or the primary care group? It can be an idea for developing a service.
- *How does the topic reflect priorities in the wider NHS, within the health authority and locally*? Some areas have a high incidence of medical or social problems, and there are initiatives from the health authority, National Service Frameworks and advice from primary care groups. Some areas may be considered to be examples of good practice by GPs (from documents such as the Fellowship by Assessment Criteria), while some are areas considered to be important by the NHS as a whole.
- *How will the practice achieve the quality improvement*? This may involve searching the literature, practice group meetings, possibly audits and surveys and the production of protocols, formularies, etc. The practice may want to invite a local expert to help at a meeting. Some areas of learning may well require a team member to attend a course elsewhere and to bring back information, or perhaps visit another practice.
- *How will the practice evaluate any improvement that is made over the next year*? This may be measurable from PACT data or through completion of an audit. It may result in completing something like the Quality Practice Award or achieving training practice status. It could be evaluated in a meeting by discussion or by developing protocols, audits or formularies.

(Extract from) practice professional development plan application form

(adapted from West Lancashire Primary Care Group)

Lead 'Education Co-ordinator':	
Practice address:	
Names of doctors:	

List size:	Training: YES/NO
Teaching: YES/NO	Premises (health centre, etc.):

Computer system and level of computerisation:
Period that this plan covers:
Names and jobs of others in the practice with personal education plans:

Topics to be covered by the plan:
- Improve patient access
- Introduce patient participation forum to practice
- Improve palliative care
- Introduce significant event audit to practice
- Audit of practice

General comments about the practice

Brief history of last year in the practice (major events/issues)
(Any major changes in the practice, people joining, any changes to the surgery, or events such as primary care groups that have had a significant impact on the practice)

Please produce a list of topics that the practice as a whole is going to learn about, develop and improve in the next year. For each topic, several areas should be addressed as outlined on the template below.

Topics for quality improvement
Topic 3 – *Improve palliative care*

How was the topic identified?

(*This may be following a discussion, analysis of PACT or other data, a patient complaint, or advice from the health authority, patient advisory group or the primary care group. It may be an idea for developing a service*)

- Discussion within the PHCT identified that we had skills deficiencies (e.g. in symptom control, use of analgesia and co-ordination of care). This followed a patient complaint from which we have tried to learn lessons.

How does the topic reflect priorities in the wider NHS, within your health authority and locally?

(*Some areas have a high incidence of drug abuse or cardiovascular disease, there are Health of the Nation targets and initiatives from the health authority, as well as National Service Frameworks and advice from primary care groups. Some areas may be considered to be examples of good practice by GPs (from documents such as the Fellowship by Assessment Criteria), while some areas are considered important by the NHS as a whole (primary care research capability, etc.)*)

- The Calman-Hine Cancer Framework[13] sets out as a priority the achievement of a better experience for patients with cancer.

How will the practice achieve the quality improvement?

(*This is likely to involve searching the literature, practice group meetings, possibly audits and surveys and the production of protocols, formularies, etc. You may want to invite a local expert to help at a meeting. Some areas of learning may well require a team member to attend a course elsewhere and to bring back information or perhaps visit another practice*)

- We shall establish links with the local hospice and palliative care team. The linked Macmillan nurse will be invited to PHCT meetings. We aim for at least one doctor and one district nurse to attend a palliative care course.

How will you evaluate any improvement that is made over the next year?

(*This may be measurable from PACT data or through completion of an audit. It may result in completing something like the Quality Practice Award or achieving training practice status. It could be evaluated in a meeting by discussion or by the production of protocols, audits or formularies*)

- We shall hold a PHCT meeting to review what we have learned over the year, and review the specific points identified in the earlier meeting referred to above.

Topic 4 – *Significant event audit*

How was the topic identified?
(This may be following a discussion, an analysis of PACT or other data, a patient complaint, or advice from the health authority, patient advisory group or the primary care group. It may be an idea for developing a service)

- Important topic which was highlighted by clinical governance baseline assessment as an area for improvement.

How does the topic reflect priorities in the wider NHS, within your health authority and locally?
(Some areas have a high incidence of drug abuse or cardiovascular disease, there are Health of the Nation targets and initiatives from the health authority, as well as National Service Frameworks and advice from primary care groups. Some areas may be considered to be examples of good practice by GPs (from documents such as the Fellowship by Assessment Criteria), while some areas are considered important by the NHS as a whole (primary care research capability, etc.)

- It is considered important by the NHS as a whole to audit significant events (both good and bad).

How will the practice achieve the quality improvement?
(This is likely to involve searching the literature, practice group meetings, possibly audits and surveys and the production of protocols, formularies, etc. You may want to invite a local expert to help at a meeting. Some areas of learning may well require a team member to attend a course elsewhere and to bring back information or perhaps visit another practice)

- By holding significant event audit meetings to discuss events and devise ways of avoiding similar events or ensuring that the positive events are used to look at methods of best practice.
- By holding significant event audit meetings regularly by 31 March 2002.

How will you evaluate any improvement that is made over the next year?
(This may be measurable from PACT data or through completion of an audit. It may result in completing something like the Quality Practice Award or achieving training practice status. It could be evaluated in a meeting by discussion or by the production of protocols, audits or formularies)

- Notes of meetings, and implementation of changes identified at meetings.

Assessment visit for PGEA approval of practice professional development plan

Practice:	Date of visit:

GP tutor/mentor/visitors:

Comments:

Recommendations for PGEA approval:
Review date:
Signature of lead GP:
Signature of GP tutor:

References

1 West M and Poulton B (1997) Primary health care teams: in a league of their own. In: P Pearson and J Spencer (eds) *Promoting Teamwork in Primary Care: a research-based approach.* Edward Arnold, London.

2 Elwyn GJ and Smail J (eds) (1999) *Integrated Teams in Primary Care.* Radcliffe, Oxford.

3 Calman K (1998) *A Review of Continuing Professional Development in General Practice: a Report by the Chief Medical Officer.* Department of Health, London (a copy of this report is on the Chief Medical Officer's website at http://www.open.gov.uk/doh/cmo/cmoh.htm)

4 Davis D, O'Brien MAT, Freemantle N, Wolf FM, Mazmanian P and Taylor-Vaisey A (1999) Do conferences, workshops, rounds and other traditional continuing education activities change physician behavior or health care outcomes? *JAMA.* **282**: 867–74.

5 Brookfield SD (1986) *Understanding and Facilitating Adult Learning.* Open University Press, Buckingham.

6 Secretary of State for Health (1998) *A First-Class Service: quality in the new NHS.* Department of Health, London (a copy of this report is on the Department of Health website at http://www.doh.gov.uk/newnhs/quality.htm)

7 Eve R (2000) Learning with PUNs and DENs© – a method for determining educational needs and the evaluation of its use in primary care. *Educ Gen Pract.* **11**: 73–82.

8 Pringle M and Bradley C (1994) Significant event auditing: a user's guide. *Audit Trends.* **2**: 20–4.

9 Pringle M, Bradley CP, Carmichael CM, Wallis H and Moore A (1995) *Significant Event Auditing.* RCGP Occasional Paper 70. Royal College of General Practitioners, London.
10 Westcott R, Sweeney G and Stead J (2000) Significant event audit in practice: a preliminary study. *Fam Pract.* **17**: 173–9.
11 Marshall MN (1998) Qualitative study of educational interaction between general practitioners and specialists. *BMJ.* **316**: 442–5.
12 Headrick LA, Wilcock PW and Batalden PB (1998) Interprofessional working and continuing medical education. *BMJ.* **316**: 771–4.
13 Expert Advisory Group on Cancer (1995) *Calman–Hine Report. A policy framework for commissioning cancer services.* Department of Health, London.

Further reading

- Wilkes D and Mills KA (2001) Using the significant event audit model and patient interviews in assessing the quality of care. *J Clin Govern.* **9**: 13–19.

Useful websites

List of directors and deans of postgraduate general practice education. From this site you can identify your own deanery and postgraduate director. Nearly all of these now have websites; http://www.rcgp.org.uk/rcgp/external/jcpt/index.asp

Dorset Centre for Clinical Governance; http://www.bournemouth.ac.uk/schools/ihcs/clingov/healthprofessionals/index.html

National Association of Non-Principals. This is one of the best sites, with a lot of information about PUNs and DENs©, and much else; http://www.nanp.org.uk/

Professional development: a guide for general practice (linked to the book of the same title); http://www.medirect.com/professional-development/

Wisdom Centre for Medical Education; http://www.wisdomnet.co.uk/index.asp

University of Exeter Significant Event Auditing Site; http://latis.ex.ac.uk/sigevent/

CHAPTER 16

A journey through cancer

Ina Murphy

This chapter puts theory into perspective. It is the story of someone who has been on the palliative care/'cancer journey'.

Having retired from teaching in my early fifties, life was jogging along quite nicely. I was enjoying pursuing my many hobbies, going on holidays and doing some supply teaching to fund this. I had always followed a healthy diet and enjoyed sport. I played a lot of golf and led a very active life. I felt fine and had no inkling of what was to come.

Something wrong?

At the end of October 1993 I visited the dentist because I had had a sore under my tongue for over a week. However, as my own dentist was on holiday I saw another one who thought it was an infection and prescribed antibiotics. The soreness persisted, so in December I made another visit to the dentist and this time saw my own dentist. She spotted a lump and was concerned enough about it to refer me to a specialist.

I was unaware that there might be anything seriously wrong, and have since thought that perhaps my dentist should have given me more information. (Last year I asked her why she hadn't told me of her deep concern, and she said that she had not wanted to worry me.)

> • Last year I asked her why she hadn't told me of her deep concern, and she said that she had not wanted to worry me.

Hospital appointments start

On 21 December the specialist informed me that I would need a biopsy and that the results would be back in a few days. At this time I was blissfully unaware that there was anything seriously wrong, as the word biopsy did not sound any alarms. (I don't why. It could have been that I was totally overcome by the whole thing, having been sent from the dentist to Selly Oak Hospital on the same day.)

Ten days later I returned for the results of the biopsy. My cousin had been planning to come to this appointment with me, but the specialist had been held up and delayed my appointment. It did not occur to me to wonder why he wanted to see me himself, rather than one of his team. So in fact I was on my own when I was told the result of the biopsy – the sore was malignant.

Bad news
Cancer: *the big C*

It had never entered my mind – it came as a complete shock. I was numb from my feet right up to my head. In this stunned state life seemed to stop, and I remember looking out of the window feeling this numbness, unable to formulate any cohesive thoughts.

The specialist was now beginning to talk about what was going to happen, but it was difficult to focus on what he was saying. (I would say that I consider it vital to have someone with you when receiving the results of such tests. At the very least they would be able to take in the information.)

> • I would say that I consider it vital to have someone with you when receiving the results of such tests. At the very least they would be able to take in the information.

'Tell anyone you have cancer and what they'll hear is that you're about to die. Why would they not? It's what you heard when you got the diagnosis, after all.'[1]

The treatment

The specialist explained that as the cancer was small, it was treatable – it was no bigger than my small fingernail. He said that I was very unlucky to have oral cancer as I was not a smoker or a heavy drinker. At 57 I was also younger than the normal age group for this cancer.

The cancer could be treated by:

• surgery
• radiotherapy
• iridium needles.

The specialist discounted the first two options and thought that the third one was the best choice. However, he wanted a second opinion, so I went to see an oncologist four days later. It was then agreed that iridium needles were the right treatment. Unfortunately, the equipment at the hospital was not in use, so I had to go to another hospital for my appointment to see yet another doctor.

That doctor explained that I would have the needles inserted into my tongue under general anaesthetic. Talking and eating would be impossible, and I would be in isolation while the needles were in place. I was told that the soreness afterwards would be indescribable and my food would have to be liquidised.

In the mean time it was back to the dentist. I had to have four teeth removed which were adjacent to that part of my tongue.

Radiotherapy

Before this treatment I tried to find out more about it but failed to do so. This left me feeling even more alone, and I did not know enough about what to expect.

> • Before this treatment I tried to find out more about it but failed to do so. This left me feeling even more alone, and I did not know enough about what to expect.

Six weeks later I had to go back to the hospital for the radiotherapy treatment. I had experienced a state of panic for days before because I did not understand what was happening. I was expecting a maximum stay in hospital of five days, but in fact I was only there for three days.

When I arrived for the treatment I did not want to be there, but the nursing staff were very good and calmed me. I wanted to run away! In fact, it wasn't as bad as I had expected, but they were certainly right about the discomfort.

Post radiotherapy

Eating normally was impossible and all of my food had to be liquidised. For six weeks I had to live on unappetising-looking food and it was a struggle to eat. The soreness made eating slow and painful. I had always enjoyed my food, and this made me determined to eat to enable me to recover (I dreamed of eating a piece of toast!). My diet was supplemented with Build-Up so that I was able to regain the weight I had lost.

In the following weeks and months I had many appointments at the hospital and outpatients with the specialist. The operation seemed to have been successful, but two months later, in April, a white patch appeared on my tongue.

Setbacks
The little white patch

The specialist was concerned about this patch, but at the second hospital it was thought to be a radiation ulcer (which I had been warned might occur).

In July 1994 I was out of pain at last and able to eat normally again, but mentally I was not dealing well with the whole thing. Since December it had been a roller-coaster of appointments and I really had not come to terms with what it all meant. I had not got over the shock. About this time I began to experience feelings of great anger. I felt angry with my body for letting me down, as I felt that I had not abused my body or taken risks with my health. I was angry that I was expected to be positive in order to fight the cancer, but what does this mean and what does it do?

- Mentally I was not dealing well with the whole thing. Since December it had been a rollercoaster of appointments and I really had not come to terms with what it all meant. I had not got over the shock.

I had to take some action about my mental turmoil, so I visited my GP, who listened carefully and said that I needed help. I told her I did not want to take drugs, but she said that was not what she was thinking about. She suggested seeing a hospice home-care sister.

This wonderful nurse was a life-saver and I am very grateful for her help and understanding. Through her visits she helped me to stabilise my mental approach and begin to come to terms with my new life now that it had been turned upside down. In one of my sessions with the nurse she suggested that I write down my feelings, and I found this very helpful. It enabled me to confront my feelings and expunge them in a way that talking about them did not. She continued to be vital to me in dealing with what was to follow.

- Through her visits she helped me to stabilise my mental approach and begin to come to terms with my new life now that it had been turned upside down.

Further soreness

In July 1994 I was asked to do some part-time teaching in the forthcoming Autumn Term, and this seemed to be a chance to help my mental recovery. It gave me a focus other than the big C, and it introduced some normality into my life. The pupils were difficult to inspire and it was certainly a challenge − I soon began to regret taking it on.

My mental state at the time made it difficult to make a rational decision. I was experiencing feelings of uncertainty and isolation. I became very emotional and sensitive to things that would not have affected me before my diagnosis. In this emotional state, I realised that I had taken a step too far in going back to teaching.

Added to all of this, at the end of the teaching day my tongue was very sore.

Another biopsy

In October 1994, a check-up with the specialist confirmed my suspicions that something was wrong. He was concerned about a hard white lump under my tongue. At first he was reluctant to do a biopsy because the tissue would not heal well due to the radiation, but eventually it had to happen and it took place in November. Seven days of waiting followed, but I guessed what the result would be. The clue came from the specialist when he suggested making an appointment when the clinic would not be so busy, so that we would have time to talk.

Another hill to climb

On 21 November I returned for the result with Pam, a friend of mine, and the news was as I predicted. The cancer was back and an operation was now required. I did not feel as stunned as the first time because I knew what it was and I was able to ask questions about what would happen. I wanted to know about the operation and what to expect afterwards. The specialist gave me the details.

- Before the surgery I would be admitted to hospital to have a PEG inserted into my stomach for feeding.
- A week later I would return for the operation. A piece of skin would be taken from my left wrist and used to replace the part of my tongue which was removed. A graft from my abdomen would replace the skin on my wrist.
- Glands would be removed from the right-hand side of my neck.
- The operation would take about 12 hours (what a shock!).
- I would be in ITU afterwards for about 24 hours.
- I would be in hospital for up to 10 days.
- My left arm would be out of use for at least three to four weeks.
- Afterwards my speech would be permanently affected.
- I would need a soft diet.
- I would need looking after for some weeks as I would be unable to fend for myself at home.

Admission

I was admitted to hospital on 1 December.

Prior to the operation there were the usual preoperative procedures. At this point, apart from the soreness of my tongue, I felt physically fit and well.

However, I was continuing to see the hospice sister who was supporting me mentally. I felt quite calm about going into hospital and had every confidence in the specialist. I felt much better informed and better prepared for coping in the future.

Before going to the hospital, I had to make preparations for when I was discharged, as I was not going home postoperatively. I remember going around the house saying goodbye to each room, wondering if I would return. My life seemed to stand still as there appeared to be no future.

> • I remember going around the house saying goodbye to each room, wondering if I would return. My life seemed to stand still as there appeared to be no future.

After the operation
In ITU

I was aware of the noise around me and the fact that I had two visitors, but I drifted in and out of consciousness.

On the ward

• I was having pain relief intravenously. My mouth was uncomfortable. It was full of saliva and my tongue felt huge, but I had no pain.
• My left arm was in a Bradford sling.
• I was allowed small sips of water.
• I communicated with pen and paper.

Progress

• Twenty-four hours after surgery, I was out of ITU.
• Forty-eight hours after surgery, the specialist told me that the graft had taken and things were going well.

Diary: Monday 5 December
I still have not had a wash. The promise of a bed bath was not forthcoming. I'm sure I would feel more normal after a wash. I did sit out in a chair for some time today.

Diary: Wednesday 6 December
Bath and hair wash at last – what a treat!

Diary: Thursday 7 December
Taken off the drip today. The dietitian came and said I was to be fed every 2 hours, but no one did it. I was told that the food to be introduced through the PEG had been ordered, but it did not happen.

I was so incensed by the lack of care that when I spotted the Ward Sister I took her to task. I don't know who was more shocked by my shouting – her or me! I questioned why doctors' instructions were not carried out for hours and why I had lacked basic care. She admitted that she had failed, and offered me a drink of Build-Up immediately.

- Four days after surgery a young nurse asked me why I was writing, and I said out loud that I couldn't talk. This was a turning point, as I had not expected this, and my speech never looked back. It was difficult to talk because of the saliva, but I persevered.
- Five days after surgery my nutrition should have been changed to taking liquid feed orally (the PEG was still to be used at night). However, this did not happen and I became very concerned that my recovery would be compromised. At that point I still had not been washed, but fortunately my cousin came and was given this task.
- Prayers were said for my recovery all over the country.

During my stay in hospital I had:

- lots of visitors and cards
- a surprise visit from relatives from Ireland who came over for the weekend to see me.

Home

After 11 days in hospital I went to stay with friends as I was not able to use my left arm. During my stay I had a plentiful supply of visitors and telephone calls – my friends always handed over the phone for me to speak for myself. This really got me using my mouth for speech again.

As for food, my aim was to get rid of the PEG as soon as possible, and my friend encouraged me to try lots of things that perhaps I might not have had at this early stage. Consequently, by Christmas Day all my food was taken by mouth (only 23 days after the operation).

Friends

The nurse at the Maxillofacial Clinic had warned me that I would find out about my true friends. I was sceptical about this. However, as time went by I found this to be true.

Some friends found it easy to support me by visiting and spending time with me. Some have found it distressing and needed my support. Others have ignored the cancer altogether.

Diary: Thursday 12 January

Sally fetched me to go to Barrie's funeral – not a very comfortable experience with her. Sally commented that I had not written a thank-you note to her son for my Christmas present. She was very put out by the fact that I had not acknowledged his thoughtfulness. The last thing on my mind! Only five weeks since my operation, my life completely changed and she didn't understand my difficulties. I feel hurt that a close friend is unable to allow me shortcomings at this time. She dropped me off a short walk away from my friend's house. I arrived back in tears, and Howard was very concerned because he'd never seen me so upset. He agreed that Sally should have been more sensitive. Fortunately for me, Howard was able to deal with my distress. I'm grateful to have good friends when I need them most.

- Only five weeks since my operation, my life completely changed and she didn't understand my difficulties. I feel hurt that a close friend is unable to allow me shortcomings at this time.

Feeling different

I do feel different – I'm not so resilient and I feel quite fragile inside.

For a long time the future was difficult, especially planning things like holidays. I felt I did not have control of my life. My confidence was shattered and although I thought that the specialist was in control, I realised that it was the cancer which was taking over.

Despite these difficulties, I knew that I had to move on and take up life again.

Strategies
Dealing with the outside world

1. I had had a lot of contact with people I knew in the days following the operation, but had not been out in public. To start with my scars were very prominent and I was afraid of public reactions, but after a visit to the supermarket I realised that my fears were unfounded. What a relief!
2. I found it difficult to talk about my experience. When I went to the clinic I didn't talk to other patients and didn't want to swap symptoms.
3. I rang the receptionist at my hairdresser's, told her briefly what had happened and asked her to tell my hairdresser. I didn't want to talk about my operation as I wasn't sure of his reaction. I did not want him to feel sorry for me. I still go to the same hairdresser and we have never spoken about it.
4. I was due for an eye test, but because I knew my optician well I decided that I could not tell him about my cancer. Instead I went to another optician, but I had to relate some necessary details. It was easier to tell a stranger.
5. I kept a diary of my dealings with life and how I felt, and I found that recording things was very therapeutic. Reading this some time afterwards made me realise how much progress I had made.

- I found it difficult to talk about my experience. When I went to the clinic I didn't talk to other patients and didn't want to swap symptoms.

Talking and speech therapy

The speech therapist visited me the night before my operation and described how I might cope afterwards. For example, I might need something to answer my phone because my speech would be impaired. She painted such a gloomy picture about the difficulties I would face that I was very disturbed by it. However, I decided that I would manage on my own, and in fact I did not need any speech therapy.

My speech gradually improved. I had to speak very slowly in order to control my tongue. Three months later I read in church.

Certain words are still difficult to say – GREEN COOK BOOK GRASS DESCRIBE CLOCK – and I am aware that I slow down when I have to say these words. Generally I have to speak more slowly than I used to, and my tongue gets tired.

Eating

Eating only takes place in the left side of my mouth, and I eat very slowly because the right side of my mouth has no sensations (the flap of skin which has replaced part of my tongue has no nerves).

My diet is much the same as before the operation, but with small adjustments. I avoid sweets, nuts, white bread and most meats (unless minced or very tender). My tongue is not able to cleanse my mouth, so I have to rinse after eating and I need to go for a scale and polish every three months.

In November 1995, I persuaded my dentist to try a denture in the lower jaw as I had so few teeth left. This improved both speech and eating.

Diary: Saturday 31 December
A year ago today I learned that I had cancer on my tongue. My mouth still feels full up (after the operation), but eating is a little easier. I ate two slices of brown bread and a boiled egg followed by a mince pie! A real achievement.

Picking up life again

It is very difficult to describe how I feel different about life. This new life is not the one I have chosen, but I have had to come to terms with it both emotionally and physically. The physical healing has been much quicker. The emotional side has caused many more problems. I am very sensitive about my health, and every pain, blemish and other symptom is *CANCER*. I feel different in that I am not as tough as I used to be, and I feel that I could shatter inside like a fragile glass.

> • I feel different in that I am not as tough as I used to be, and I feel that I could shatter inside like a fragile glass.

In order to help me to come to terms with this new life, I have kept myself busy and have become involved with many new interests.

These activities have included the following.

1   Helping children with special needs in a primary school (where I was a governor).
2   As a result of my contact with the Hospice Sister I was asked to speak to fourth-year medical students about cancer and its effects, diagnosis, treatment and mental upheaval. I have given these talks regularly. A bonus here was that I heard a consultant psychiatrist speak to the students about mental problems in cancer patients. This made me realise I was not alone.
3   At the request of the specialist I have spoken to dentists at the West Midlands British Dental Association about oral cancer and its effects.
4   I have helped a friend to build up a business by telephoning potential customers.
5   I was Secretary of the Ladies Section of the Golf Club for three years. I had to teach myself to type! I am now helping out with the County Juniors.

Despite initial difficulties in planning holidays, I now go away more frequently than before. My experiences have changed my attitudes to life and brought out dormant qualities and talents. For example, I had not realised how determined I am.

• My experiences have changed my attitudes to life and brought out dormant qualities and talents.

With the future uncertain, I am now more likely to take the opportunities that life offers me as I continue to pursue old interests and find new ones on my journey to recovery.

• With the future uncertain, I am now more likely to take the opportunities that life offers me as I continue to pursue old interests and find new ones on my journey to recovery.

A cancer scare

In June 2000, I was confronted by my fears again when my dentist found a white lump on my tonsils. The specialist did not know what it was and sent me to an ENT specialist. I had a few worrying days waiting before finding it was nothing more sinister than trapped food, which he removed.

I have been able to be reassured by the follow-up appointments with the specialist. He is a good listener and generous with his time, and he has always answered my questions. I know that I can phone up for an appointment if I am worried. This access is very important. I would like to say how supportive the specialist and his team have always been, and how helpful this has been to my recovery.

> • He is a good listener and generous with his time, and he has always answered my questions. I know that I can phone up for an appointment if I am worried. This access is very important.

Reference

1 Diamond J (1998) *C: because cowards get cancer too.* Ebury Press, London.

Index

Page numbers in *italics* refer to boxes, figures and tables.